Sweet Surrender

Christian 12-Step Recovery from Food Addiction

Revised and updated edition

Includes testimonies of people living free
from yo-yo dieting and overeating

Pam from Auburn, MA.

Dedication

To the yo-yo dieter, the frustrated, the confused,
the sick-and-tired-of-being-sick-and-tired overeater.
May the Lord use our testimonies to help and
encourage you.

SWEET SURRENDER

Contents

SWEET SURRENDER

Acknowledgements

To Jesus: Thank You for Your never-ending goodness, mercy and grace.

To my son, Joe, my right-hand-man, technical advisor, prayer partner: None of this would have seen the light of day without your kind heart and incredible patience in teaching me basic computer skills, and your ability to design fulloffaith.com was a gift from the Lord. Thank you, Joe and Stacy, for your constant love, encouragement and assistance.

To my 13-year old grandson, Caleb, for his helping me tweak the final draft.

To Pastor Douglas Geeze and the people at Faith Church in Auburn, MA: I will be forever grateful. You brought the Word of God to life for me and my boys, and you taught us that Jesus and His church love real people in the real world.

To Hilary from the UK, thank you for your ongoing help and encouragement in co-facilitating the *Full of Faith* ministry.

To Sanda from CA, thank you for giving me your time and gifting me with your God-given talents in editing this edition of *Sweet Surrender*.

And to the *Full of Faith* team of leaders and all the participants, thank you for being a part of this ongoing mission. It is an answered prayer.

Foreword

I am not who I once was. Thank the Lord! Who would have believed that my heart, my mind, my attitude and my behavior could be changed? God knew.

> Long ago, God promised that he would "comfort the broken hearted...captives will be released and prisoners will be freed...he will give beauty for ashes, joy instead of mourning, praise instead of despair." (Isaiah 61:1-3, *New Living Translation*)

When I read this passage, I believed God's Word, but I now know that it's personal. God says, "for you, too, Pam!"

In 2000, God asked me to write my testimony. He said, "Build it and they will come." I was asked to build a bridge between the church and the 12-step rooms for food addiction recovery. Many people in the church needed (and still need) to hear about food addiction, and many people in the 12-step rooms needed (and still need) to hear about Jesus.

I was obedient and published the first edition of *Sweet Surrender* on November 28, 2013. My history is the same, but through the hard knocks of experience, I made some changes along the way that I will portray in this edition. This edition also includes testimonies from others who have been set free from yo-yo dieting and overeating by actively

1

participating in the *Full of Faith* ministry.

Full of Faith Ministry

Mission Statement

Full of Faith, Christian 12-Step Recovery from Food Addiction, exists to touch the heart and mind of the person who struggles (or has struggled) with compulsive or addictive eating. With a disciplined way of eating and life-style changes based on biblical truths, God's love and grace bring transformation and restoration.

Ministry Team

Pam Masshardt, author of *Sweet Surrender, Christian 12-Step Recovery from Food Addiction*, started her ministry, *Full of Faith,* in the year 2000. On July 23, 2019, she celebrated 31 years of freedom from yo-yo dieting and overeating, maintaining a 75-pound weight loss. She abstains from sugar, flour, natural and artificial sweeteners, trigger foods, plus amounts. *Sweet Surrender* and www.fulloffaith.com reveal the intimate details of her testimony.

Pam and her team of ministry leaders advocate for the education and awareness of food addiction - a physical, emotional and spiritual malady for the compulsive and addictive eater. The Food Addiction Institute (www.foodaddictioninstitute.org) gives evidence that supports their claims.

Outreach

Full of Faith is an on-line ministry from *Sweet Surrender* and www.fulloffaith.com.
We offer help and encouragement through Facebook private groups, phone meetings, ZOOM video conferencing and one-to-one communication. All are welcomed - Christians and people who are not sure how they feel about their relationship with God.

We use the Bible, The Big Book of Alcoholics Anonymous, and *The Twelve Steps for Christians* to encourage life-style change. Leaders share their personal experience, strength and hope in experiencing a sweet surrender. There are no dues or fees for membership.

Vision

Testimonies will proclaim how God has used *Full of Faith* as the catalyst to share the good news that Jesus and a biblical approach to recovery from yo-yo dieting and overeating brings freedom to those struggling. The message of hope will be heard around the world. People will get set free. News will spread and more will be set free.

SWEET SURRENDER

Introduction

Dare to Dream

(flashback to 2013)

Blessed are those who hunger and thirst for righteousness, for they will be filled. (Matthew 5:6, *New International Version*)

Over the Rainbow

Sitting on the edge of my seat, I nervously awaited my cue to approach the podium. Pastor Doug was speaking on addictions and all the things that make us feel separated from God. I was invited to share my story as a testimony of God's ability to heal broken hearts, minds and bodies. "Lord, help me," I prayed with nervous, yet hopeful and trusting anticipation. I came from rags to riches. I was once a frightened woman stuffed to the brink of explosion with too much food in her belly. Day after day, I attempted to diet, as I flipped through magazines looking for the latest "cure-all," or I laid limp on the couch in utter despair after yet another binge. Now I was, by God's amazing grace, qualified to speak about freedom from yo-yo dieting and overeating. Who would have imagined?

Short moments seemed like interminable hours. I wondered what I would say. I prayed hard. Alone I could do nothing, but with God, all things are possible. "Please, Lord, speak through me. If it is Your will, use me to touch one heart, to help one hurting soul," I urgently cried out to God. When the time finally came, I took a long, deep breath and walked up to the podium.

"Hi, I'm Pam, recovering food addict and codependent.* On July 23, 1988, I turned my will and my life over to the care of God as I understood Him. I said 'Yes' to life and let go of a self-destructive habit that was killing me physically, emotionally and spiritually. With the help of God, I stopped overeating one day at a time, and God has been faithful to carry me from there."

My words seemed to float into the sanctuary like precious bubbles. I saw compassionate nods and tear-streaked faces as the glistening of hope surrounded wounded hearts and spirits.

Many years ago, God met me while on my knees. I didn't want to die, but didn't know how to live without food, my best friend. Among my half-eaten boxes and bags of food, I remained slumped in hopelessness day after day, week after week, month after month. I saw a glimmer of hope in the 12-steps, but I was naturally defiant and strong-willed. It was years later when I finally admitted defeat.

*Codependent is the term used to describe a person who is recovering from unreasonable enmeshment in the lives of others.

Reach for a Star
Sweet Surrender is my story. It is my innermost thoughts and feelings as I trudged along the rough and rocky road toward recovery. Through the help of like-minded people, I learned how to live without excess food, and I found a God who was real and available. He touched my heart, soothed my restless spirit and continued to help me each new day.

[Jesus said] ...even if you had faith as small as a

> mustard seed you could say to this mountain,
> 'Move from here to there,' and it would
> move. Nothing would be
> impossible. (Matthew 17:20-21, *New Living*
> *Translation*)

Prayer changes things, and God can make what seems impossible, possible. He asked me to write the first edition of this book in the year 2000. An ordinary woman, wife, mother, and daycare provider with a high school education was asked *by God* to share the gifts that He had given to her. At first, I was flabbergasted with the thought of it, but I knew God was calling me to higher ground, so I said, "Okay, if You want me to do it, You'll get me through it."

At times of incredible struggle, disappointment, and discouragement, I wanted to say, "This is too hard," but I heard, "He who began a good work in me will be faithful to complete it."

Please, God, anoint these pages beyond mere words. Whether you are a full-blown food addict like me, or you are struggling with an uncomfortable feeling around a little extra food or a few extra pounds, we share common ground. From experience, I know what it feels like to be overweight, and I know what it feels like to finally hit, then maintain, goal weight. Beyond physical health and a thin body, I have been blessed with peace of mind and a heartfelt desire to know God in a personal, life-changing way. I pray that for every reader. Use this book, Lord, if it is Your will, to touch the hearts and minds of people who are thirsty for more - more God, more health, more peace.

Chapter One

Realization—The Truth of the Matter

I lie in the dust, completely discouraged...
(Psalm 119:25, *New Living Translation*)

Perfect People and Other Myths

Growing up, I used to have a wonderful fantasy that I would marry an athletic-looking man and we would live in a comfortable house with a beautiful, well-manicured lawn in a pleasant neighborhood. In the evening, I would be the perfect wife listening attentively to my husband and making pertinent comments as we discussed the events of his day. Soon we would be blessed with a child or two. I would be the perfect mother cooking nourishing meals and making sure my children were always happy. He would be the perfect father, happily changing diapers when they were babies and playing sports with them when they were older. They would be clean, well-behaved, and lovable. They would be perfect children. They would be one of our biggest delights. Every day our lives would be filled with bliss and happiness.

Unfortunately, somewhere on the road of life my fantasy took a wrong turn. I met Carl and we married. He was not the athletic-looking man of my fantasy world, but he was intelligent with a nice sense of humor. However, this intelligent man that I married had a terrible flaw. He was addicted to alcohol. When he started drinking, he could not stop. Unfortunately, and unbeknownst to him, he also married a person with a terrible flaw. I was addicted to food. I was not a woman who overate occasionally, but a woman with a serious problem. Once I started eating, I could not stop. These addictions, along with some other instances of life's burdens, came frighteningly close to destroying our lives.

We did buy a house, a bona fide handyman special. It had no well-manicured lawn, but it was in a decent neighborhood, and it was ours. We did have children, two beautiful boys, Daniel and Joseph. They were my heart's delight. My whole world revolved around my children. I had succumbed to the idea that the perfect husband and the perfect house were unrealistic aspirations. Yet, I held tightly to the illusion of wonderful, well-mannered, perfect children. It was my earnest desire to be the perfect mother.

We plodded along reasonably well until 1980 when Carl lost his job after seventeen years of employment. It was not "personal." The company relocated to another part of the country. This was a time when business in America was suffering and new jobs were practically non-existent. Carl knocked on doors looking for employment while I sat at home worrying and stuffing myself with food.

Carl became a "jack of all trades." Installing rugs, working construction, delivering knives, he did whatever work he could find in hopes of gathering enough money to pay the ever-increasing pile of bills. Tending bar was his favorite. He met like-minded people and escaped from the concerns of the world. Many of these casual acquaintances helped him find lucrative leads to other money-making positions. We lived from paycheck to paycheck on the wings of a halfhearted prayer.

Occasionally, my parents and my stepsister, Lorri, helped

us by supplying food, shoes, or clothing for the boys, but Carl was a proud man. He didn't take handouts easily. It was a tough place for me. Not knowing where to turn, I ate more food. At this time in our lives, fear and financial insecurity robbed us of any peace we may have had in our home.

One day, my cousin, Linda, suggested we might help each other. Her infant daughter, Angela, needed a babysitter and I needed money. It was a welcomed solution. I helped Carl with our floundering finances while I continued to stay home with our children. Thus, my daycare career began. The news spread quickly. Soon I had a house full of children and a new goal: I would be the perfect parent/daycare provider to *all* the children in my care. It was yet another impossible dream. Just like my goals of a perfect husband, home and children, my estimation of excellence was more than unreasonable. My goals were unreachable by human standards. Therefore, anxiety and frustration consumed me. When my workday was over and my boys went to bed, I collapsed on the couch and ate junk food.

Early in life, I learned how to handle emotional turmoil. My mom would say, "Have a cookie, Pammy, that will make you feel better." It was like an old wives' tale, a myth for sure. I did not feel better after eating a cookie, a box of cookies or ten boxes of cookies. After eating the first few cookies, which was my usual intention, I lost sight of reason and my rampage would begin. Time after time, despite determined efforts to control my overeating, I gorged myself with food. With each bite, I sank lower into a pit of despondency. Whatever happened to my dreams of perfection? My hopes were lost in a deep sea of despair and a high mountain of food.

Cinderella Weighs in at 202 Pounds

One unforgettable morning, I crawled out of bed in my usual daze at the demands of my screaming year-old son, Joe. On the way to the door, I caught a glimpse of my reflection in the mirror. It was not a pretty sight. I went back to the nightstand to grab my wire-rimmed eyeglasses to take a closer look. My too-small nightshirt clung tightly to my bellowing hips. My thighs jiggled like Jello and looked like cooked oatmeal. As I walked toward the mirror, I saw my long dark hair straggled around my puffy face. Tears welled in my eyes. What had happened to me?

My mother once told me a story about her best friend's mother. She was obese. Every time this mom came to school, the young girl cringed with embarrassment, almost mortified. The child often ignored her mother's presence and sometimes, even worse, she denied that she knew her at all. *Ouch.* My heart fell to the floor with a loud thud. I saw that mother in MY mirror. *I refuse to be that mother. My diet starts today, no ifs, ands or buts. My children will never know that pain.*

I greeted Joe's wailing with a feeble attempt at a smile. I was trying to be a "good" mom. As I rescued him from who-knows-what, his outlandish behavior stopped. Joe was just like me. He wanted what he wanted when he wanted it. The moment he opened his eyes, no matter what time it was, day or night, he expected to be released from the captivity of his crib, and he expected my full attention. I rarely slept because I refused to let him cry. God forbid, he might feel unloved or abandoned.

I scooped him up and headed back to my room to face the dreaded task of getting dressed. Rescuing my worn-out jeans from the pile of dirty laundry, I sucked in my gut to zip them up one more time. I couldn't face buying another size twenty. I dismissed the thought because today I was going to start my diet. I would soon be wearing smaller sizes. Determined to follow my food plan, I set forth to conquer my world. I kicked the laundry pile against the wall and thought about making the bed. *If anybody were to see this room, I'd die.* Joe and I went downstairs to the living room. I plunked him in front of the television set. *Thank you, God, for Sesame Street.*

Taking a moment to breathe and stretch, I felt the oh-too-familiar wave of discouragement and groaned. My overeating was not my only problem. Our home was old and in sad repair. It wasn't the condition of the house that made me shudder, it was my irresponsibility with the cleaning—I didn't know how to clean, and I didn't care enough to learn or to do the work. My kitchen floor needed scrubbing, the living room needed vacuuming and the dust was piled high on the furniture. The laundry stayed in mounds here and there. Outdated magazines, papers and old mail covered the coffee table. Other things were tossed under the couches to give an appearance of a respectable dwelling. I didn't wash windows. It didn't even occur to me that people did seasonal cleaning. Basically, my house was run-down and unkempt, like me.

I looked at the clock and moaned again. My first daycare child was scheduled to arrive at 6:00 A.M. I have fifteen minutes to get myself breakfast before I begin my workday. Just then, the door opened and in walked Jessica. Forcing a smile, I welcomed her, but inside I was angry. I wanted to eat my breakfast without worrying about more children. Obviously, that didn't happen, but it was okay. Jessica happily joined Joe in the living room and I continue my mission.

I rummaged through my desk searching for my nutritionist's most recent suggestions. The sheets of paper were tattered and worn from the number of times I had played with them, the number of times I had attempted to follow the plan, and the number of times I had thrown them in the air disgusted with my inability to succeed. This time was different. *Please, God, this time has to be different.*

Whenever I started a new diet, I felt obligated to update my weight chart. Hard as it was to see the consequences of my behavior, I went into the bathroom and removed every stitch of clothing before I stepped on the dreaded scale. I held my breath, as if that made a difference. I removed my eyeglasses and my rings. *Please, God, I pray that I didn't do too much damage this time.* Gathering my courage, I took the step. When I saw "two hundred and two," tears of unbelief welled in my eyes. I double-checked the reading. It was the same. *Yikes...I have gained ten pounds in two days. I am so sick. I need to stay on this diet today.*

I practically knew the food plan by heart. Breakfast was a serving of oatmeal, a cup of milk and a fruit. I quickly prepared and ate my breakfast. Other children were due to arrive at the daycare. Dan stumbled down the stairs, joined Joe and Jessica in front of the television and said, "I'm hungry. Mama, I want something to eat." Just like me, he thought it was time to eat as soon as his feet hit the floor. I gave him some graham crackers to share with his friends as they arrived.

Around 8 A.M., I grilled some English muffins to serve with breakfast. Dan ate the centers, but refused to eat the edges. Usually those were mine. I delighted in eating the leftovers. After all, my mother used to tell me that children were starving in Africa, and it was my obligation to eat them and not waste food. Somehow that made sense to me. *I am not going to eat the leftovers today. I don't need their food. I have a new diet. I can do this. I need to do this today.*

In daycare, meals and snacks are scheduled at regimented times. Snack time came quickly (10 A.M.). I tried to keep it simple by serving toast and juice, but the committee in my head started negotiating. *I could have a piece of toast if I eliminate the grain from lunch. I will be fine. Okay, I'll have one dry piece of toast.* However, one piece was not enough. The next piece had peanut butter and jelly on it. *I'll skip lunch. I WILL be fine.* In a heartbeat, my somewhat composed disposition took a nosedive. Threads of anger bubbled within me. I started snapping at the children for no good reason. Distancing myself with a "don't look at me" sneer, I tried to overcome my fear of failure. *What is wrong with me? I can't even diet until lunch!*

Lunchtime was approaching, and I, naturally wanted more food. Was I hungry? Who knows? *I already ate lunch at snack time. Please, God, help me. I can wait until dinner. I will barbeque a luscious T-bone steak, bake a potato and steam some vegetables. That is certainly a hearty meal. It will be wonderful.* Anticipation kept me focused for the rest of the afternoon.

I fed the children lunch. This time I threw the leftovers in the trash and smiled. *Wow, that was good.* I felt like a hero. *I can do this. I will be fine.* Later, we baked corn muffins, and I made myself a cup of coffee instead of eating even one crumb. Patting myself on the back, I was pleased. *I am really good. I can do this.*

Dinnertime came. My mouth watered as I envisioned the delicious dinner I had planned. It was like a love affair; I could not wait to be alone with my lover—the food. In order to thoroughly enjoy my "date," I cooked dinner for the family first. Carl volunteered to entertain the boys while I cleaned up their dishes and ate my meal. I took advantage of the offer, served my bountiful feast on fine china, and sat at the head of the table all by myself. I felt like royalty. Eating one precious bite at a time, I spent nearly half an hour alone with my best friend, food. *This is great. I love this diet. I could do this forever.*

As I washed the rest of the dishes, my mind raced to my next move, *oh no, my food is gone for the rest of the day. What am I going to do? I could watch television, but without food, it wouldn't be fun. I suppose I could review this new diet and plan my meals for the week. It would be better to think about the diet than to think about eating more food.*

Around 7 P.M., Dan and Joe were tired, and Carl's patience was wearing thin. In a matter of minutes, he was more than annoyed. It was my responsibility to protect the boys from his anger, but as usual, I joined him, yelling in an attempt to keep some semblance of a loving home life. What a tangled web! I yelled to keep him from yelling. Frustrated, I swished the boys off to bed.

It was my routine to read books and sing songs until the boys were asleep, so, as usual, I read their favorite stories and sang some soothing melodies. This time, however, my head was in the clouds; I was thinking about food. In time, the children settled down, and I joined my husband in the living room. *What can I do now?* Anxious and annoyed, I told my husband I wanted to catch up on some reading and suggested that he go to bed early. Because he was exhausted, Carl willingly agreed that he could use some extra sleep and went to bed.

My pride kept me from telling Carl I was dieting again. I cannot count the times I was convinced I had finally found the answer to my food problem in some new and improved diet. It never changed anything. I would start off gung-ho only to fail once again. The embarrassment and shame were devastating. *This time will be different. I will prove that I can diet and succeed once and for all. I'll show him.*

Last Supper and Then Some

Everything looks different at night. The ghosts and goblins come out of the woodwork, so to speak. That night all of my troubles were magnified. My burdens were too heavy to bear. My husband had problems, my children had problems, and I had problems. I wanted to fix everything and everybody. *Life should be easier.* I sat alone with no answers, no comfort, and no food. I continued to dream. *Where is my fairy godmother?* I longed for a place, some fantasyland, where all the streets were paved with gold, and everyone felt loved. Oh, what a glorious place that would be! Fairy tales are for princesses, not for me. I lived in the real world with real problems. Gloom and doom accompanied my somberness. *Poor Pammy, poor sad*

Pammy.

Smothered by my insecurities and my fears, I remembered my mother's words, "Here, Pammy, have a cookie. That will make you feel better." *Maybe I could have a piece of fruit. The diet suggests two pieces a day, but three could surely be considered reasonable. Don't you think?* The committee in my head concurred. Quickly, I scurried into the kitchen and found a beautiful apple. I grabbed my cutting board, my favorite paring knife, and my special fork. Bringing my treasure to the living room, I artistically cut it into dinky, bite-sized pieces and slowly, carefully relished every mouthful. *That was okay. Apples are a healthy snack, only 60 or 70 calories. It takes 3,500 calories to gain a pound. I am still a "good" girl.*

Now what? I was hungry, or so I thought. I definitely wanted something more to eat. I pondered my options. It was only 8:40 P.M. The grocery stores were still open. *What should I do?* Marching to the kitchen, I began my hunt. Slowly and thoughtfully, I opened every cabinet door. My resolve to diet was waning. Fortunately, the cupboards were relatively empty, as food didn't last long in my house. I quickly ate whatever I bought. I felt relieved and considered going to bed; then a light bulb went off in my head. *Uh-oh, I'm in trouble now.*

Carl had some goodies put aside in his desk. I had promised not to touch them. He used to get rip-roaring mad whenever I ate his food. Once he even threatened to buy a lock and key to protect his stash. *I can't eat his stuff.* My history went before me. I would eat his food time and time again, and then I would fabricate elaborate excuses for the missing sweets. Most often I would plead, "Someone stopped by, and I *needed* to offer them something." Other times I would say, "I gave the children your goodies as a special treat for exceptional behavior." I had to lie because the truth was unacceptable, even to me. At the time of the heist, I would lose touch with reality. I became compelled. It

17

was almost like an out-of-body experience.

Even though I knew it was wrong, I once again inspected Carl's hidden supply of chocolate kisses, peanut butter cups, and chocolate covered cherries. *I could eat a peanut butter cup and replace it tomorrow. He won't even know.* Snatching my treat as one might steal a kiss from a married man, I ventured back into the living room where I could fully enjoy this mouthwatering sensation. I slowly removed the wrapper. With anxious anticipation, I used my special knife to cut it into many tiny, bite-sized pieces. I slowly, lovingly devoured each morsel. *I love chocolate. I r-e-a-l-l-y love chocolate.* I was drawn back to Carl's hidden reserve and helped myself to the remaining splendor. *I'll start my new diet tomorrow. I didn't follow the plan today anyway. I had better go to the store and replace Carl's food.*

Gee, what else should I eat tonight? Chocolate chip ice cream, raw cookie dough and chocolate fudge frosting — maybe just a little of each? I could use some cookie dough to bake cookies with the daycare children tomorrow. It will be the craft project of the day and my excuse for shopping tonight.

Enthusiastically, I hopped in the car and headed to the market to buy replacements for Carl's candy. I also bought a bag of chocolate kisses for me, plus a half-gallon of ice cream, a stick of ready-made cookie dough, and a can of fudge frosting. On the way to the checkout line, I grabbed a box of chocolate chip cookies for the boys. As I drove out of the parking lot, I rummaged through the bags searching for my beloved chocolate kisses. I downed six as I sped home, one mile down the road.

Gathering my bags from the car, I tiptoed into the house hoping everyone was still sleeping. I listened to the silence for a brief moment, but I was anxious for my tantalizing delights. I dashed to the kitchen and modestly scooped a reasonable portion of ice cream into my favorite bowl. I sliced four pieces from the stick of cookie dough and placed a dollop of frosting on each one. *I'm only going to have one bowl. I'll eat it slowly and r-e-a-l-l-y enjoy it. Normal people eat a bowl of ice cream and a few cookies as a snack. I have certainly had enough junk food today.*

Sitting in front of the television, I savored every bite. *That was so good. I want some more food. I guess it was stupid to think I could stop after one bowl. I am so sick. It has been less than two minutes and I need some more food.* Disgusted with my inability to control my eating, I hung my head in shame and retreated to the kitchen once again. I retrieved the half-gallon of ice cream from the freezer, the rest of the cookie dough, and the wonderful chocolate frosting. I started eating directly from the containers, frantically concerned Carl might wander downstairs and notice my outrageous behavior once again. After all, my love affair with food was my precious little secret.

Halfway through the frosting, I felt physically sick. My stomach felt as if it might explode, so I got a bucket in case I threw up. *What is wrong with me? I don't want any more food, but I cannot stop eating.* I quickly dumped some filthy cigarette ashes into the partially eaten container of frosting, closed the lid, and threw it in the trash. *Okay, good-bye frosting.* Somehow, I managed to eat the rest of the ice cream and polished off the cookie dough feeling a little worse with every bite.

Suddenly I had an idea. Maybe I should make myself throw up. Months earlier, a friend told me how to induce vomiting. She said it helped her to stay thin. "Put a spoonful of mustard in a cup of water; drink it, dash for the bathroom." Her words sounded ridiculous to me until today. *If I can make myself throw up, I can eat and not get fat. That sounds pretty good to me.* No matter how hard I tried, it didn't happen. I tried shoving my finger down my throat. No luck. *I can't even throw up right. I am such a loser.* I gave up and started to cry. Moments later, I was face first on the bathroom floor sobbing uncontrollably. *What is wrong with me?*

With my heart pumping wildly in my chest, I thought I was having a heart attack. My stomach felt like a water balloon ready to burst. *I am going to die. I should wake Carl up and go to the hospital. On second thought, no, I can't do that, if I have to tell him all I have eaten, he'll think I'm crazy. I am crazy.* I dragged myself into the living room and passed out on the couch until Joey startled me with his crying once again. It was 5:30 A.M., and I needed to get ready for a new day.

Back to the kitchen I went. My binge foods were gone without a trace except for the boys' cookies that were sitting untouched on the counter. Poor cookies! They never stood a chance! *I'll just have a couple.* I started with two. Two became four, then six, then eight. In a matter of a few seconds, the whole row disappeared. Anger welled within me. Disgusted, I threw them on the floor and stomped them to death. As I discarded the cookie crumbs in the trash, I noticed the discarded can of frosting from the night before. Before I could stop myself, I retrieved it, scraped off the ashes and ate the disgusting frosting. *I am really sick! Why can't I stop eating?*

I had now lost all control. Anything edible was mine. I frantically concocted make-believe cookie dough by mixing together a little flour, some sugar, a blob of butter, and a dash of vanilla. I ate it raw. I then found some old nuts, jimmies, chocolate chips and the like. Desperate and afraid, I sprayed oven cleaner on a batch of something. Convinced it was poison, I finally had a reprieve.

Minutes later, I found an old pie crust mix. I proceeded to make pinwheels by spreading a little butter, a sprinkle of cinnamon and a spoonful of sugar on the dough. It took barely fifteen minutes to bake. As I waited, I found a stash of brownies in the freezer. I gnawed on one while the others defrosted in the microwave. I also ate raw pudding mix moistened with a little hot water. Had I not blacked out here, I'm sure my rampage would have continued.

I cannot remember everything I ate on this one occasion out of many. It was volumes; enough to put on fifteen pounds in three days. I was sick and tired, but try as I might, I could not stop overeating. I didn't want to die, but I didn't know how to live. *Help me, Lord.*

Weighting in the Wilderness

"Ring-around-the-Rosy, a pocketful of posies. Ashes, ashes, we all fall down." I traveled around the same mountain doing the same things over and over again expecting different results. Diet after diet, I tried and failed. I could not stop overeating. My doctor sent me to a nutritionist who gave me a nutritionally sound food plan that sounded great on paper. Unfortunately, it was the same dilemma leading to another frenzy of compulsive overeating. I felt helpless, alone and afraid. The definition of frenzy in Webster's Dictionary explains it all: temporary insanity.

I was obsessed with being thin and spent hours at the library seeking new approaches to losing weight. On the way home, I would stop at a store to pick up my last splurge. Any diet started with a binge. The Grapefruit Diet, The Cabbage Soup Diet, The High-Protein, Low Carbohydrate Diet, The Aids Diet Candy Regime, Atkins, The Slim Fast Diet, I tried them all. Nothing worked.

A special occasion, the high school reunion, the summer vacation or a holiday celebration always managed to put me into a tailspin. To me, if you looked good, you were good. Fat was ugly and unacceptable. I would put my best foot forward and try, *really try*, to diet faithfully. With my eyes on the calendar, I often dropped a few pounds. However, as soon as the big day arrived, my usual eating regime returned followed by more compulsive overeating and more pain. My weight rose with each event.

Desperate for help, I considered weight loss programs. I invested considerable amounts of money in Weight Watchers, Diet Workshop, Gloria Stevens Fitness Center and other programs offered at local hospitals and medical centers. History repeated itself over and over again. I committed to a program, attended the meetings, and stepped on the scale (being careful to wear my lightest clothing). The next day was a free-for-all. For one day, I ate whatever I wanted. Then I would diet all week preparing for my next class, the weigh in and my reward of a day off. It was a vicious cycle.

Initially I experienced success, but I would soon begin to rationalize and justify my need to stay home: *My husband and children need me, and we cannot afford to be spending money on frivolous things.* Each time I left a program and stopped going to meetings, I made a solemn promise to continue to diet. Time after time, I tried. Time after time, I failed. Embarrassed, frustrated and confused, I could not understand why these techniques worked for so many people but not for me. *What was wrong with me?*

Chapter Two

Acceptance —
Real People in the Real World

They will rebuild the ancient ruins and restore
the places long devastated; they will renew the
ruined cities that have been devastated for
generations. (Isaiah 61:4, *New International
Version*)

Live and Learn

In the beginning was the word and the word was "food." It
was not logical, fruitful or fulfilling, but the message had
been passed from one generation to the next: "Food will
make you feel better." Children learn to live from their
parents, just as their parents learned to live from their own
parents.

The "ham story" explains this idea of blind adherence to
our own upbringing, whether or not it makes sense. A
mother and daughter are in the kitchen doing some
preliminary preparations for a family celebration. As she has
always done, the mom cuts the ends off the ham and puts it
in the oven. The daughter asks, "Mommy, why do you do
that?" She shrugs her shoulders and without much thought,
she says, "Because that's what my mother does." The
daughter goes into the living room where the other family

23

members are mingling and addresses her grandmother. "Grandma, why do you cut the ends off a ham?" She answers almost immediately, "Because that's what my mother does." They turn to her mother, three generations down the line, for the answer. With a shy, almost embarrassed smile, the great grandmother says, "My roasting pan is rather small; I have to cut the ends off the ham, so that it will fit it into my pan."

Too often we don't question the why and wherefore of things. It is like using autopilot in an airplane. The pilot rests in the fact that the plane has been programmed properly. What is the programming that guides each of our lives? What values have we been taught through the years? What messages have we inadvertently heard that have shaped who we are today?

When we open our eyes and see the truth, the whole truth, we have an opportunity to change. Cutting the cords to our self-destructive past performances, we grow confident in our God-given abilities and strengths. People don't know what they don't know. We live and learn.

Goldilocks and Her Two Brothers

Throughout my childhood, my family was the typical mother, father, two boys and a girl scenario. As respected members of the community and local church, we lived in a nice little town in a quaint little house in New England. My mother was my hero. She was kind, caring, and considerate; she was my best friend. Although she was not obese, my grandmother, all my aunts, and most of my cousins were severely overweight. Food was the answer to any problem in my family.

My twin brother, Ricky, with his small frame, light complexion, and blond curly hair, resembled Mom. The family humorists say that when we were in my mother's womb, I must have squished poor little Ricky in the corner. "That's why he's so scrawny." Ricky was a sensitive

24

child who struggled academically. I somehow felt it was my job to take care of him. I would often try to "feed him happy." Whenever food was served, I'd take mine and then ask for his. I was known to say, "Ricky will have a cookie." Little Ricky was not like me; it was a bother for him to eat meals, and snacks were a waste of time. I loved my little brother but felt rejected when he said, "You eat it." Even so, I was happy to have more food. It was my consolation prize.

John, my older brother, was reasonably proportioned with light wiry hair and glasses. We had little in common. John was an intellectual who, in my eyes, lacked compassion. It hurt when he sang, "Tubby, Tubby two by four, couldn't get through the garden door." I was not exceptionally overweight as a child, but when he sang, I felt huge, unacceptable, and unlovable.

Dad was a charmer and the love of my young life. He was tall, dark and handsome. At six feet, three inches and two hundred forty pounds, Dad towered over Mom. He seemed invincible, yet he was like a teddy bear, soft and cuddly. I was certainly Daddy's little girl.

As far back as I can remember, Mom controlled our sweets by distributing allotted snacks. I politely ate my small, respectable bowl of ice cream or my one or two cookies with the family. Later, with no one in sight, I ignored the rules. Holding my spoon in one hand, the half-gallon of ice cream in the other, I ate. Be it a box of cookies or a pan of brownies, it didn't matter. I never intended to eat the whole bag or box of anything, but I was compelled. I could not stop. Panic and despair followed each episode. Constant battles warred in my head. To eat or not to eat, that was the question!

Halloween was a given: I ate. Pillowcase in hand, I was on a mission. When the porch lights went out, we hurried home to empty our bags on the living room floor. *I cannot eat my brothers' candy this year. If I got caught, I would be mortified*. Mom told us to eat one piece a day. I tried. I *really* tried, but my candy was gone in a day. Unable to stop myself, I would then sneak into my brothers' bags and ate theirs. The love of food won over rational thinking every time. I kept looking for logic as I asked repeatedly, "What is wrong with me?" I never did find the answer.

I was fat, in my opinion, and I had two left feet. Even though I hated being fat and clumsy, I delighted in my family's reaction when I skinned my knee or bumped my head. My grandfather would buy me candy and goodies every time I got hurt. Once I tripped and fell on a piece of glass, cutting my elbow right to the bone. I waited anxiously for Grandpa's response. He gave me one dollar, a lousy dollar! I felt separated from Grandpa's love. To me, sugary treats looked like love, smelled like love, and felt like love.

Family celebrations were wonderful. I happily volunteered to assist Mom anytime we entertained guests in our home. My delight was wrapped in thinking about, preparing, and eating the food. I licked the spoons, cleaned the bowls with my fingers and sampled the results. My job as a young teenager was arranging the pastries on platters. All the imperfect pieces, or the ones with slightly burnt edges, were mine. I loved being behind the scenes; no small task for me. I had a plan and a goal: keep everyone happy, feed them, and feed me.

By evening, I would feel unacceptable, undesirable and unlovable. Therefore, cleanup was certainly better than talking with the people or hiding in a corner hoping to remain unnoticed. I took advantage of all the leftovers and ate off the guests' half-finished plates. I was stuffed to the brim dreading the next day when my new diet was to begin.

Humpty Dumpty Sat on a Wall

"Wake up, Pammy. It's time to get ready for church." I jumped out of bed and started rummaging through my closet. *What am I going to wear? I wish I were thin. I wish*

I hadn't eaten so much food yesterday, but it was a party. Everyone eats at parties. Please, God, help me stay on my diet today.

Dressed in my brown hide-it-all skirt, I sat and listened to another sermon on God's love. *I wonder what the snack will be at coffee hour? God, help me to stay on my diet today.* Week after week, we sat in our family pew, the one invisibly marked with our name on it, listening to a similar message: if you follow the Ten Commandments and live a good life, all will be well. God was watching over his children. Heaven is a nice place where people go when they die. *When is the pastor going to say, "Amen"? I am getting hungry.* As soon as the usual greetings and casual chit-chat ended, I was out the door investigating the food choices at coffee hour. I politely ate my two cookies. Not satisfied, I decided to rethink my plan. *Maybe two more and I'll skip my bread at lunch. I'll say, "I'm getting these cookies for Ricky."* Still wanting more, I grabbed a few and slid them into my purse for later. *Monday is a better day to start my diet anyway. Nobody starts a diet on Sunday. Today I'll eat. Tomorrow I'll diet.* If people noticed my behavior, at first, I might have cared a little, but then it didn't matter. I simply needed more food.

Dad and John continually implied I would be happier if I were thin. I heard, "You have a pretty face. It's too bad you cannot control your weight." Lovingly, John referred to me as pleasantly plump, which meant I was nice, but fat. Nearing my first year of high school, John became disgusted with my attempts to diet. He said, "You can't lose weight. Why bother? I'll give you twenty-five dollars if you lose twenty-five pounds." He had no intention of losing his precious twenty-five dollars. He was arrogant and insensitive, but I was stubborn and headstrong. *I'll show you. Don't tell me I can't do it.* We were both amazed when I won the prize. I enjoyed a thin body for a few weeks, or was it days?

I was a mystery to Mom and Dad. Even with all of their encouragement, I continued to fail. I appeared strong in public, but behind closed doors, I ate. I was an expert in hiding my boxes, bags, and containers of food. Discouraged, embarrassed, and humiliated, I continued to cry, "What is wrong with me?"

Humpty Dumpty Had a Great Fall

Hope soared as I entered my junior year of high school. The peer pressure and my interest in boys created a positive mindset. I was able to maintain a reasonable body weight for the first time in my life. I felt attractive. I found some friends, dated some respectable boys, and participated in social events typical for my age. Just when I thought my life was finally heading in the right direction, my world fell apart.

It was the summer of my senior year when Mom went into the hospital for a hysterectomy. The doctor said it was a common surgical procedure. There was no need to worry. Five or six days later, the bomb dropped. *What do you mean she's dead? You said it was a common, everyday operation. What am I going to do? Mom was my best friend. Why did she have to die? It's not fair. It's not fair. It's not fair.*

Alone in my room, I cried. Mom's words resounded in my head, "Have a cookie, Pammy, that will make you feel better." Buried deeply in grief, my self-esteem diminished, and my self-control evaporated. Alone and afraid, I did my best to hold the house together as chief cook and bottle washer. My dad and brothers tried their best to be supportive and encouraging, but it was tough. We all had our own struggles to face.

My dieting dilemma returned with an added quest: find my perfect mate. After graduation from high school, I opted for a full-time job as a secretary at a well-known distribution center. It seemed that my sole goal in life was to get married

28

and have a lot of children. I envied my married friends who were starting families. They looked happy and content. They had a purpose. I needed a purpose.

I wandered through life searching for the answer to the question, "How can I get thin." *If I were thin, I would be happy. Someone would love me. I would get married and have my babies.* I spent my time in diet programs, exercise studios, health facilities, singles clubs, church socials, bars and the mall hoping to bump into someone special. No partner could be found. As the months sped by, I sunk lower and lower into a pit of despair.

Twinkle, Twinkle Little Star

With endless typing, dictation and filing, daily work was exceptionally boring. *I need something to eat.* It was around two o'clock in the afternoon. I pumped my handful of quarters into the candy machine and hit the button five times. I tucked the candy into my purse and proceeded to the ladies' room. *I can't let anyone see me eating five candy bars. What would they think of me?* Hiding in one of the stalls, I quickly unwrapped and devoured all five in a matter of minutes hoping no one would interrupt my self-indulgent spree. Distraught with yet another episode of overeating, I went back to my desk and waited for the day to end. After work, I visited the mall hoping to gain a new perspective.

As I was walking into the front entrance, a fine-looking young man with beautiful brown eyes and light wavy hair approached me. He introduced himself and asked if he could talk to me for a minute. His name was Gary. My heart started beating. *Is this the one? Is this my perfect mate?*

It wasn't a minute into the conversation when I realized he was a "holy roller," a zealous spokesman for God. I told him I was fine; I went to church, or I used to go. I didn't drink. I never smoked. I never did drugs. I was a nice person.

He opened his tattered Bible and read some

verses. Mesmerized, I heard that everyone needs
God. Everyone makes mistakes. God sent His only Son,
Jesus, to die an awful death on the cross to pay the price for
my sins. He asked a simple question, "If you died tonight,
are you sure you are going to heaven?" I thought for a
minute and replied, "All people go to heaven, unless they are
really bad, and God probably forgives them, too. God is a
forgiving God." Gary looked at me in amazement. With a
waning confidence by now, I nervously proclaimed, "I am a
good girl." I then proceeded to blurt out some kind and
loving things I did for people. He stopped me short and said,
"You cannot earn your way to heaven."

I was getting annoyed. I spouted off in a brewing huff,
"How do YOU know you are going to heaven?" He didn't
react to my brash attitude. His calm demeanor stayed firm
as he explained his position. "I acknowledged my need for
God, admitted I was a sinner and asked God to forgive me. I
know from the Word of God, The Bible, Jesus died for my
sins. I invited Him into my heart. He is my Lord and
Savior."

Gary showed me some verses in the Bible: God's Purpose:
Romans 5:1, John 3:16; Our Problem: Romans 3:23, 6:23;
Our Powerlessness: Proverbs 14:12, Isaiah 59:2; The
Solution: 1 Timothy 2:5, 1 Peter 3:18a, Romans 5:8; Our
Choice: Revelations 3:20, John 1:12, Romans 10:9;
Assurance: Romans 10:13, Ephesians 2:8-9.

After some heartfelt twinges, I asked him what I needed to
do to get right with God. He said it was simple. "If you
believe what I have told you, tell God how you feel." I sat
and pondered my choices. In a few brief moments, I knew
what I needed to do. Timidly, I welcomed Jesus into my
heart and my life.

"God, I have made lots of mistakes in my life. I am
sorry. The Bible tells me that everyone makes mistakes; it is
the human condition. No matter how hard I try, I cannot be

perfect. That's why I need you, Lord Jesus. Please help me to know and do Your will today. I thought that everyone went to heaven when they died. I now see Your message of hope is for believers. I believe that the Bible is The Word of God. I believe that You died so that I could live. Your Holy Spirit will guide me and help me in this life, and I will see You face-to-face one day in the next. Thank You, Lord, for this amazing gift. Amen."

Thirsty for more information about God, I went to the religious bookstore with eager anticipation and purchased a beautiful, leather-bound Bible. A woman in the store suggested the King James Version. I had my name boldly imprinted on the cover. I knew then my life would never be the same again.

Alone in my room, I opened my precious new Bible. I started reading...*Adam and Eve, Cain, Abel and Seth—what do they have to do with my life?* I glanced ahead, flipped through some pages. It was like a foreign language to me. Confused and disappointed, I put the Bible on my bedside table and continued my search for the perfect diet and the perfect mate.

Jack and Jill Went Up the Hill
Years went by. Dad married one of the secretaries where he worked. John married a girl he met in college. Ricky married a girl from the lake where we had our summer home. Still alone, I sat in my apartment and wept. *"What is wrong with me?"*

Thank God for my job. Five years as the secretary to the purchasing agent at a large well-known distribution center proved I had some worth and value. I loved my job and I did it well.

"Pam, did you hear about the new job?" The word spread quickly about a new position in the warehouse of two hundred fifty men and a few women. *If you want a man, go where the men are.* It was a division of the Personnel Department, a one-girl office. I was overly qualified, but the company agreed to move me laterally. I wanted that job.

I had constant contact with men. I was the woman to see for any personnel problems or concerns. My title was Administrative Assistant, which meant receptionist, payroll clerk, insurance claims coordinator, and secretary to the warehouse manager. It was the perfect job for me.

Carl was the working supervisor of the Parcel Post Department. "Hi, Carl, how's it going today?" I said. He was friendly, but not my type. He was small, kind of gruff-looking, and divorced with four children. We found common ground by the copy machine. I had problems. He had problems. In time, we became dependent on each other. It only made sense that we should marry, so we did.

Carl knew my heart. We had talked about children for hours before we were married. I would be an at-home mom. He liked being a dad. Due to complicated circumstances, it was difficult to fulfill his role as a father to his four girls, and I was too self-centered to understand my responsibilities as stepmother. Our first son, Daniel, was born in 1980. I soon discovered being Mom was not as I had expected. Nothing ever was. It was hard work. Carl drank and I ate through our problems. Daniel needed a playmate, so Joseph was born in 1983.

My parenting skills were those I had adopted from my own experiences growing up. "Here, Danny, have a cookie. That will make you feel better." It was the "don't feel" answer to any problem. I taught my boys well. They were invited to my eating frenzies, respectably called a party. We planned a celebration for one reason or another and bought the appropriate party supplies, lots of food. Still intending to enjoy only one piece or bowl, we began the festivities.

It was fun for the first five minutes. The boys ate their

treats and wandered off to play, leaving me alone with the food. One slice of cake was never enough. I slivered a little from one side, slivered a little from the other, eventually devouring the whole thing. One spoonful of ice cream led to two, to three, and finally to consuming the whole container. I was sick and tired of being sick and tired, but I could not stop overeating. I tried. God knows I tried day after day. My overeating splurges evolved into a way of life, coupled with frustration, hurt, disappointment and rage.

My poor children, God bless them. They had a loving mother one minute, when my diet was going well, and a screaming maniac the next, when my diet was abandoned yet again. I was physically and emotionally exhausted, hopeless, and full of despair.

My binges became more often and more severe. Raw chocolate chip cookie dough, chocolate fudge frosting and a half-gallon of ice cream, that's where I began. Anything edible followed. I ate until the food was gone or I passed out, whichever came first.

Desperate and fearful for my health and life, alone in the confines of my mind, I begged God to show me a way out of my misery. *Help me, Lord. I do not want to die and abandon my children. There has to be more to life than this. I am begging you, Lord. Help me, please.*

I didn't know many verses in the Bible, but I remembered Mom wearing a necklace with a mustard seed charm. She told me the story about faith. She said, "If you have faith as small as a mustard seed, God can help you."

> ...*Anything* is possible if you have faith... I *do* have faith; oh, help me to have *more!* (Mark 9:23-24, *The Living Bible*)

Jack Fell Down

I felt like a single parent, fully responsible for the children and our home. Carl worked most days and nights. One day he came home all excited. His words gushed like a babbling brook, "Baby - we always called each other "baby"- Baby, I got a job. It's our dream-come-true. I'll be working at the utility company. For six months it will be tough, but after that we'll be fine." *Yahoo, we are finally on our way to happiness. Thank you, God.* We rejoiced and were glad.

The months rolled by, but nothing really changed. He still worked many hours, and came home only to collapse and pass out on the couch. Even though his new job was flexible, and he could have come home after work as early as 11:30 A.M. sometimes, he never did because he didn't want to be around the "bunches of children hanging on the furniture." That's how he described the daycare.

In time, I had had enough. I needed a break or even a divorce!

"Dad, can the boys and I come stay with you for a few days? I am leaving Carl." Sad as the situation was, my father welcomed us with open arms. *I love my daddy. I am still his little girl.*

Outside of close family members (Dad, my stepmother and my stepsister, Lorri), no one knew I was troubled, not even Carl. I had been taught to keep secrets. My mother would say, "We don't talk about our problems; we don't show the neighbors our dirty laundry." The simplified message was, "Shut up. Keep the peace at all cost."

Carl returned home from a deep-sea fishing trip to find a note on the table. "We're at Dad's. I won't be back." Shocked and dismayed, he was breathless. I blamed all our problems on him and his drinking. I thought that if only he were sober, we would have that storybook family life like Ozzie and Harriet, and I wouldn't overeat. I would be fine if he would just stop drinking.

Carl asked if I would help him get sober. He said, "Baby, come home for three months. If I take even one drink, you can leave." I loved him. I hated the alcohol. It was a fair deal.

And Broke His Crown

A banner hung from the blackboard, "The Twelve Steps." My eyes were drawn to the words, "Came to believe that a power greater than ourselves could restore us to sanity." *Sanity...what's that?*

With apprehension and fear, we attended a recovery group for alcoholics. I went along to support and encourage Carl's newfound hope of sobriety. We found some seats in the dreary, smoke-filled room. I glanced around at our counterparts. It was certainly a mixed bag of people, mostly regular folk like us.

Men and women shared bits and pieces of their lives: the good, the bad and the ugly. I heard some amazing things that first night. "Alcoholism is a debilitating sickness. It is progressive and can be fatal. It affects the whole family." I cried and I laughed. Somewhat baffled, I knew these people were talking directly to ME, and I marveled at their honesty. *These people are showing me their "dirty laundry." They have secrets like me. I am not unique. Carl is not the only addict in this family.*

One woman was talking about having "just one glass of wine with a meal. After all, it was a celebration." She could not stop. I could relate. One piece of birthday cake or one cookie and stopping, never happened for me either.

The man dressed in black was discouraged. I nodded in agreement when he said, "What is wrong with me?" He tried to do controlled drinking. "I'll only drink beer and no hard stuff," "I'll only drink after 8 P.M.," "I'll dilute the alcohol in milk." He failed every time.
"When a normal person discovers that he has a flat tire, he

35

calls the garage. When an alcoholic gets a flat, he calls suicide prevention." *Yup, that's me, too, extreme in everything.* A calm sense of peace came over me. I felt hopeful. Carl was sober. Maybe I could win over my addiction, too. "It is just one day at a time." *Tomorrow I'll begin my diet.* The meeting ended with the Serenity Prayer.

And Jill Came Tumbling After

One day, a good-intentioned friend visited us and gave Carl a book that he referred to as "The Big Book." He said that he was an alcoholic and this was the "Bible" of the program that worked for him. I grabbed it before Carl could say a word and said, "Can I read it? I *know* that I am an addict. Sweets are my alcohol." Our friend released it to me with a smile. However, Carl looked at me as if I were crazy. He rolled his eyes and said sternly, "Food is not like alcohol." Under my breath I mumbled, "I'll show you." I was serious and confident God had given me my answer.

As soon as I was alone, I read Bill's story. He was the founding father of *Alcoholics Anonymous*, an interesting man, mixed-up and unbalanced like me. I recognized my warped, exaggerated imagination, my lost reasoning, and my lack of self-control. *I am an addict. Addiction is addiction. I know God wants me to be happy and healthy. Diets don't work. Okay, God, help me to apply these principles to my food problem.* "The Twelve Steps are the map of the program," echoed in my mind. Making it personal, I replaced the "we" words with "I".

Step 1: I admitted I was powerless over food, that my life had become unmanageable. *No doubt. I think about food day and night. I try to control myself, but I cannot stop overeating even though I know bingeing and starving is harmful and possibly fatal. I don't want to die, but I don't know how to live.*

I pondered **Step 2: Came to believe that a power greater than myself could restore me to**

sanity. According to Webster's Dictionary, sanity is freedom from mental derangement, being reasonable and sensible. *I need sanity in my life.* A memory of my mother flashed before me. She was teaching me lullabies one restless night. "Jesus loves me this I know for the Bible tells me so." *I believe in a power greater than myself. I believe in God. Yes, most assuredly. I will never forget my experience in the mall years ago, and I know God brought me to Alcoholics Anonymous to teach me how to live without sugar. I will learn to live as a recovering addict.*

Step 3: Made a decision to turn my will and my life over to the care of God, *as I understood him*. *Okay, God, I believe you want me to be free from my addiction. I will stop eating my "alcohol." I will stop eating sugar-laden junk food.* The program emphasizes one day at a time. I made the decision: no sugar for one day.

My day began with a healthy breakfast: a grilled bagel, an egg and a banana with my pot of coffee. I felt fine for about ten minutes; then my head started to spin. By noon, I was eating anything and everything once again. *I am not an alcoholic. Food is different, not like alcohol or drugs. People who drink excessively act inappropriately, trip and stumble, slur their words, pass out on park benches. No one even knows I have a problem. Besides, how bad can it be? Every church has sweets and treats mingled into celebrations, meetings and social affairs. People are asked to enjoy the food. To apply the steps of Alcoholics Anonymous to my problem is foolish thinking. Carl is right. I am crazy. I was grasping at straws and employing desperate thinking. Food is not like alcohol. There must be another answer for me.*

Chapter Three

Surrender —
Addiction is Real, Debilitating and
Ultimately Fatal

He lifted me out of the pit of despair, out of the
mud and the mire. He set my feet on solid
ground and steadied me as I walked along.
(Psalm 40:2, *New Living Translation*)

Sparks of Light

Carl was recovering one day at a time. It was a miracle
happening before our eyes. He learned how to live without
alcohol. I watched him with amazement as I continued my
search. The days and months rolled by. Hopeless and
helpless, I was as desperate as the dying can be.

In lieu of eating yet another bite of whatever, I grabbed
the Sunday newspaper and scanned the classified section for
feasible options. A 12-step program caught my
eye. Nervously, I dialed the number. The phone rang for
what seemed like fifteen hundred times. Finally, a soft-
spoken woman answered. I asked if she would send me the
diet. I explained that meetings might not work for me. It
was hard getting out of the house, leaving the kids and all. I
remember her gentle chuckle as she replied, "This program

39

does not promote any food plans." She graciously offered to send me some information. Two days later, my newcomer packet arrived, along with a questionnaire. My very first inventory looked something like the one below. (*15 Questions*, Copyright l986. Reprinted by permission from the publisher).

1. Do you eat when you're not hungry?

Yes, I eat for other reasons, including anxiety, frustration, boredom and the like.

2. Do you go on eating binges for no apparent reason?

Some of my binges are not planned. Most of my binges are not planned. I make a decision to have a small, reasonable portion (two cookies or a candy bar). My one or two pieces become four, then six, then eight until the whole bag or box disappears. I know in my head I need to stop. I want to stop, but I continue to raid the cabinets searching for more food. Feeling like a failure, I think, "I might as well continue to eat today. Tomorrow I will start my diet." I pray for the ability to stop as I consume whatever I can find, the better-quality foods first. Then whatever appeases my appetite for the moment. Nothing satisfies my hunger. I go into a trance. I have absolutely no control.

3. Do you have feelings of guilt and remorse after overeating?

I feel like a failure. I should be able to control my eating. Why can't I stop eating? It makes no sense to me.

4. Do you give too much time and thought to food?

I think of food all the time. I am forever trying to control my diet. Plus, it seems all our fun times are planned around food. For me, special foods are associated with different events—ice cream, fried dough and fudge at the beach, S'mores and popcorn by the fire at a campground, or hot chocolate with marshmallows and doughnuts at a winter outing.

5. Do you look forward with pleasure and anticipation to the time when you can eat alone?

I love to eat alone. When my husband has to work late or has an evening meeting to attend, I set up my plan for the night. I wait until the boys are in bed and begin my rendezvous with the food: an elaborate dinner and an extraordinary dessert. More times than not, it leads into an explosive free-for-all binge.

6. Do you plan these secret binges ahead of time?

Whenever I find a new diet, I need a day to prepare. I eat all the things that I will never-have-again. I also give myself permission to enjoy special days or a holiday season or wonderful vacations.

7. Do you eat sensibly before others and make up for it alone?

I can make a good impression by eating reasonable portions in front of people. It is embarrassing to be overweight and overeating. In a stressful situation or even a celebration, my mind is rushing to the reward coming. Alone, I can truly enjoy my food.

8. Is your weight affecting the way you live your life?

Dad refers to me as "happy go lucky," but the truth is I am not happy. Most assuredly my weight is affecting my life. I should not feel so distraught. I have a nice home, a husband who loves and supports the family and two wonderful children whom I adore.

Carl and I have had our difficulties, but we are okay. I know it is God's will for me to be a responsible, loving parent and a caring wife. I am successful most of the time; however, I could be kind and loving one minute, when I am in control of my food and having a "good" day on my diet, and then on a "bad" day, I am like another person—some eccentric lunatic. My poor husband and children are ignored, or worse, I get angry. I start banging cabinet doors and complaining about everything and everybody.

By the grace of God, I have the ability to save most of my overeating until late evenings. Then I can refrain from hurting the people I love. I am alone with my food. The only victim for my abusive thoughts and actions is myself. Outside the home, when I am obliged to attend a social affair or a sporting event, I sit somewhere hoping to remain unnoticed. I am ashamed of my size and my lack of grace. I waddle when I walk. I fear people judging me, as I am judging them—fat is ugly. Thin is beautiful. I would prefer staying home where I am safe and secure in my private little world.

9. Have you tried to diet for a week (or longer), only to fall short of your goals?

I have been successful at times for a week or more, but never long-term. I give up and go back to my normal eating habits. Maybe I need to accept myself as a fat person. Some people say I am big boned. I see overweight women on television who are happy. They say, "Big is beautiful." I don't agree. Thin is beautiful. It is my hope, my dream, and my vision to be thin.

10. Do you resent others telling you to "use a little willpower" to stop overeating?

I want to yell and scream, "I AM TRYING TO USE WILLPOWER." I get angry and embarrassed when people can see my problem.

11. Despite evidence to the contrary, have you continued to assert that you can diet "on your own" whenever you wish?

I keep trying, but I haven't been able to diet, with or without the help of diet programs, in a very long time. Something is wrong with me—in no time, my mind strays off the goal, I lose sight of my vision and I overeat.

12. Do you crave to eat at a definite time, day or night, other than mealtime?

I think of eating all the time, but the desire is more

*intense mid-afternoons, when the children are napping, and
late evenings, after my boys are settled in bed. I like to eat
when I finally sit down and relax.*

13. Do you eat to escape from worries or trouble?

*I do not intentionally eat to escape from my troubles, but
I do find myself overeating when I am worried. It seems to
be a natural reaction for me.*

14. Have you ever been treated for obesity or a food-related condition?

*I have gone to doctors and nutritionists for help. Each
time I was given a new and improved diet, and I was
instructed to practice self-control. Maybe I need a
psychologist—a doctor to help me handle my
emotions. Maybe then I could control my overeating.*

15. Does your eating behavior make you or others unhappy?

*My eating behavior makes me very unhappy, and my
family is affected by my low self-esteem. I am hurting
myself, but I cannot stop. I don't know how to stop. I know
God loves me and wants me to be happy. Why do I keep
overeating when it makes me so unhappy? What is wrong
with me? Something is definitely wrong with me.*

Shine Little Glow Worm

Passing the test with flying colors, I qualified for the title,
"Compulsive Overeater." It was an easy mark, A+, no doubt
in my mind. I could have asked more questions or attended
a meeting listed in the packet of information, but instead I
harbored resentment and anger. For months, I blamed my
upbringing, my husband, and my circumstances for my sorry
state of affairs. Mixed-up and confused, I continued my
efforts to control my diet. I continued to fail, and, in time, I
gave up.

Sobbing into my pillow after yet another awful day of
overeating, I made the decision to attend a meeting "for

curiosity's sake." Being an instigator and a saleswoman by nature, I dragged my cousin and my best friend along for the ride. They were eating buddies and diet-minded like me. It was an easy sale, a miracle cure. We all wanted to be thin, but had no idea how to stop overeating. Anxious for help, we found a meeting the next day. It was conveniently located at a local church hall.

I welcomed Saturday. With the sun shining brightly through the beautiful blue sky I gathered the troops and drove to the meeting. We walked into the building and followed the signs for the meeting location. As always, I led the way. At the far corner of a huge hall, people were arranging metal folding chairs in a circle. One of the stout women sauntered across the room to greet us. I assumed she could tell by our sizes that we were looking for a diet group. We introduced ourselves and settled into some seats close to the door. She smiled politely and whispered, "You have come to the right place."

There were maybe twelve to fifteen men and women in the group, mostly young and middle-aged adults representing a wide scope of shapes and sizes. Some were bone thin, some were grossly obese and some were normal sized, appearing pretty healthy. *That's what I want. I wish that I could be normal sized and healthy.*

The meeting opened with the Serenity Prayer. My mother loved that prayer. She would mumble it whenever she needed help. It was like a quick release switch to soften life's dilemmas.

> God grant me the serenity
> to accept the things I cannot change,
> the courage to change the things I can,
> and the wisdom to know the difference.
> (Reinhold Niebuhr)

Peace, acceptance, courage and wisdom, how do I apply

that to my overeating? I listened intently as the men and women talked about the changes that had occurred since joining the program. The most prevalent message was, "I stopped compulsively overeating by practicing the program. Just like the recovering alcoholic stops drinking, I do it one day at a time." I was intrigued. My friends, on the other hand, were not pleased. I could tell they were disenchanted the moment we walked into that musty church basement. They wiggled in their seats, looked at me, looked at their watches every few minutes, and looked at me again. Their unspoken words were written across their scowling faces, "Why did you bring us here?"

The meeting closed with the Lord's Prayer. I gathered some pamphlets from the literature table, and we left without saying a word to anyone. On the way out the door, my companions laughed at the "sick people" and vowed never to return. Feeling embarrassed by my own sickness, I remained silent. I needed to return. My life was at stake.

Glimmer, Glimmer

At home, I read and reread my pamphlets. In my dreams, I fancied myself as one of those thin, healthy-looking women. Although I could not imagine life without occasionally overeating, I was ready to attend my second meeting. This time, I traveled alone. As I entered the church hall, a kind-looking and rather plump woman recognized me from the week before. She smiled meekly and said, "Welcome back." I felt an immediate bond as her sad eyes met mine. She told me about her week, and I told her about mine. We were both out-of-control eaters. I did not intend to tell her what I did with food, but as she told me her tragic tale, it was easy to tell her my equally disheartening food-induced woes. We were like sisters, two peas in a pod. We smiled in hopeful anticipation as the beautiful speaker-of-the-day began her talk.

She was not an eloquent speaker by any means, nor did

45

she look happy. As I saw it, she was just like me, crazy, always thinking about food and her weight; however, there was a difference, a big difference: she was thin and was no longer overeating. The woman said, "Get a sponsor who has what you want and ask how she is achieving it." She looked good to me. I wanted to get thin. Therefore, after the meeting, I bravely approached her. "Please, can you help me?"

She peered at me, acted rather perturbed and said, "Are you sure you are ready to give up sugar?" Evading the question, I explained that I was a newcomer to the program, but I was an informed dieter. I asked, "Could I follow a diet from Weight Watchers or Diet Workshop?" Disgruntled, she said either diet could work *if* I carefully refrained from sugar. I overlooked her unpleasant attitude and agreed sugar was certainly a problem for me.

After an anxious moment and a sigh, she apologized for her inconsiderate behavior and explained that she had a full plate. Many people called her during the day at pre-arranged times to commit their food. She seemed to force a smile and said, "Okay, we'll try it. Call me at 8 A.M. tomorrow, and tell me what you are going to eat for the day."

Driving home, I felt as if a giant boulder had been lifted off my shoulders. I had someone who was helping me. I actually had a group of people helping me. I was not alone anymore. The sun felt warmer, the sky seemed bluer, and life seemed better. Then a revelation hit me. It was a spiritual awakening of sorts. Twelve-step programs work because people share from the heart of experience. What a simple concept. *Thank you, God. My sponsor person might not be the most pleasant woman in the world, but whatever she is doing works for her. That's good enough for me.*

As I was nearing home, I wondered what to tell Carl. I was afraid of his reaction to yet another dieting scheme. He had already witnessed so many new diets, so many hopes, dreams and failures. My fear kept me silent, and I reasoned that he didn't need to know the details anyway. The proof would speak for itself. I quietly rummaged through my books and decided on a diet. I jotted down my intended plan for the next day. It was a funny state of mind; I was happy to have found my answer, but I was afraid. *No more cookies, no more cakes, no more cookie dough or frosting?* It only made sense to eat all the things I would never be able to eat again. I was kissing my goodies good-bye, so to speak. Although I knew I would feel physically full, it seemed okay this last time. My life was about to change.

Starlight, Starbright

The next day, I awoke eager to begin. I called my sponsor and told her what I was planning to eat for the day. Program jargon confused me. The word "abstinent" was in every sentence. I asked, "What does it mean to be abstinent?" "It is simple," she said, "Abstinence is refraining from compulsive overeating. When people say they have been abstinent for a year, it means they have followed their diet every single day for a whole year." That amazed me. How could anyone go a whole year without sugar? *That would be a miracle for me.* She went on to say that a sponsor is the person who helps you get started. She tells you what to do to achieve abstinence.

I was ready to receive my instructions: "Read a daily meditation book for addicts," and call other people who are in program. Ask them how they stay "out of the food." It was all new terminology. "We don't eat one day at a time." I asked, "What do you mean you don't eat?" She said, "We eat what we plan and nothing else. Some people do a "301 meal plan of eating," three meals a day with nothing in between, except water or black coffee, one day at a time." My sponsor believed in a less restrictive approach. Any diet without sugar was fine. Nutritionally, it made sense to me. We were off to a good start.

"Get a pencil and paper," she commanded. "I want you to

jot down some telephone numbers. Keep them on the side of the refrigerator for easy reference." This woman knew lots of people and all their telephone numbers by heart. "You need to hear about compulsive overeating and how to stop when you get too hungry, angry, lonely, or tired." She said, "We need to halt. Remember that word." The phone call concluded with one more question. "Can you make a commitment to attend a meeting every Saturday morning?" I told her I would try. "It might be difficult because my husband works a lot, and I have two small children." She understood and told me to go if I could.

It was Sunday morning, around 9 A.M., when I hung up the phone. Amazingly enough, everyone in the house was still sleeping. Although I felt leery calling strangers, I had agreed to call one person sometime during the day. I took advantage of the free time and called the first person on my list. The first call went well. I felt compelled to call the next person and continued until I had called every person on my list. It was a new fun experience. People wanted to talk. They seemed happy to have gotten my call. I sat in awe at the thought of the strangers who wanted to help me. All this advice was free. People helped people just because people had helped them.

Somehow, I stayed on my diet for days, weeks and months. My weight dropped steadily, and I gathered strength, wisdom, and understanding as I avoided sugar one day at a time. I learned to redirect my compulsive nature to helping other sick and suffering overeaters. I made phone calls, encouraged people, and never said, "I can't help you." I had the answer: people helping people. Without sugar, it was easy to diet.

All That Glitters is Not Gold

It broke my heart to see many people walk into our meeting never to return. I had been given an extra measure of compassion for the discouraged overeater. My family and job sat on the back burner at this stage of my life. When the phone rang, I talked. I was on a mission to save *all* the compulsive overeaters who needed help. I faithfully attended the Saturday meeting and shared my success story each week.

Being bold and outspoken, my reputation went before me: "She's a know-it-all." It fit me. My big-shot attitude kept me hopping from sponsor to sponsor. I did not listen well. I already had the answers. I felt that I had done my homework. My personal dieting experience, plus the oodles of books about nutrition that I had read, made me an expert, or so I thought. I was certainly a whiz at food exchanges and calories.

As I continued in the program, my harshness softened, and I became a desirable sponsor. Knowing about nutrition was helpful in leading people to a healthy food plan. The list of people that I sponsored was long, too long. Coming from extremely low self-esteem, I reveled in being good at something.

I gradually forgot about taking care of myself. I was so busy helping everyone else that I didn't have time to talk about me. At one point, I was relieved when my "sponsor of the week" ate and decided to leave the program. I made the decision to sponsor myself. Why not? I was successful and I was thin. My sick thinking told me that my time would be better spent sponsoring other people. I was fine.

Without a sponsor, it was easy to make exceptions to the rules. I ate more than my plan allowed, usually additional protein, potato or rice. I forgave myself each time and decided I could not be perfect, nor did I want to be.

People talked about different food plans. Some people were successfully doing a food plan that sounded dreadful to me. It was called the "The Gray Sheet." I supposed that the original plan of eating must have been printed on a gray sheet of paper. It was a food plan that eliminated all grains. It certainly didn't appeal to me. I liked my grains. I couldn't imagine life without them. I ate oatmeal for breakfast; at lunch and dinner, I ate rice cakes, baked potato, or some rice. I avoided bread because it was too fluffy. However, somewhere along the line, I made the decision that diet bread would be okay. It was an easy option. In time, I went to a nutritionist for more ideas. She suggested that a bagel or a muffin might add some variety. We discussed my goal to avoid sugar. She understood how junk food could be detrimental to my health but convinced me that bagels and muffins were healthy exchanges.

One day I said, "Okay, I will buy some corn muffins." I had avoided sugar for nine months, but how much sugar could there be in one corn muffin? Empowered and confident, I felt the health factor would benefit me. It would be fine. I knew how to stay on my diet. I was abstinent from sugar, I was thin, and I looked good. *I can do this. A corn muffin is a healthy food. I'll be fine.*

The big day came. I ate my corn muffin, and I felt like a hero. Three days later, I bought six corn muffins and ate them in the car on the way home from the store. I was shocked at how fast the familiar pattern of compulsive overeating, followed by stringent dieting, returned. Embarrassed, I attended fewer meetings. Quietly sitting in my chair, my face revealed my pain. I had lost my status and become a seeker once more.

I tried and tried to follow the same diet. I could do it for a few days, sometimes a week or a month, but then I would binge once more. Two years passed while I searched for the answer. People at the meetings told me that I had fallen off my pink cloud. Others told me I was doing more research. I was doing more pain, more compulsive overeating. People often say, "There is nothing worse than a belly full of food and a head full of program."

Follow the Yellow Brick Road

Somberly, I waited for the meeting to begin. Empty and alone, I hung my head in shame. *What is wrong with me? I cannot make it through one day on my diet.* A tear trickled down my cheek. *Lord, please show me the way. I am so tired.* The day before my mother died, she was heavy-hearted and discouraged. She looked to the sky and reminisced. A comforting verse came to mind.

> Jesus said, "Come to me, all you who are
> weary and burdened, and I will give you rest."
> (Matthew 11:28, *New International Version*)

Please, Lord, help me. What do You want me to do?

A radiant young woman volunteered to lead the meeting. Hope glistened in my heart when she described her transformed life. My heart skipped a beat when she explained her food plan, absolutely no sugar *or* flour. She boldly proclaimed, "My food plan is weighed and measured. Sugar *and flour* are no longer options for me."*

*[The refinement process of whole grains into flour increases the absorption rate of these foods into the bloodstream. Only a tad slower than sugar, flour affects the serotonin levels in the brain. That's why we feel like sleeping after a binge of highly refined carbohydrates. Serotonin acts like a tranquilizer, a painkiller and an escape from life.]

I froze for a moment in shock as my brain struggled to comprehend that ghastly thought. *No flour?* I cringed, and my heart ached. My mind spun in search of logic. I wanted to deny the validity of such drastic measures. *Come on, Lord, flour, too? Flour is healthy. My nutritionist told me breads and pastas are good foods.* My future was grim. I could not imagine life without flour - my muffins, my bagels, my "healthy" foods. I asked for an answer, some other answer, any other answer.

God whispered in my ear, "Can you do it for one day?" I stopped grumbling. *Maybe, just maybe, recovery is more complicated than I thought. Flour could be addictive. Sugar is certainly a problem for me.* It was a miserable thought, but I was tired of living a miserable life. Gloom and doom had followed me for a very long time. This woman had celebrated five years of abstinence. She was thin *and* she was happy. She had a calm delight, an aura of godliness, and I desperately wanted that peace.

She volunteered to sponsor one new person, one *serious* person. She only helped people looking for *serious* recovery. I was desperate and I was tired of doing things my way. It didn't work. I remembered my first spiritual awakening months before. 12-steppers share from the heart of experience. This profound experience birthed my second spiritual awakening; *recovering* food addicts not only weigh and measure their food, but they avoid sugar *and* flour.

My first phase in program was a diet. I had listened to Weight Watchers logic. I had gotten thin, looked successful, and felt good for a while. A diet is only a diet. Food addiction relates to specific foods known to set up cravings in the body of an addict. God wanted me to understand the severity of the disease and the power of His help.

Jesus Gave Me a Sunbeam

"Please, let me be the one." Her twinkling eyes met my pleading spirit. She said, "That would be wonderful." My heart rejoiced. *Thank you, God.* It was as if a beam of sunshine landed on my shoulders and radiated its warmth all the way to my soul. My life changed as my wellspring of knowledge disappeared.

I surrendered my will, my wants, my intellect and my perceived know-how to her. She understood the intricacies of food addiction. She set the guidelines beginning with my diet. She gave me the basic plan that had been passed down the line of sponsors. The bottom line was absolutely no sugar and flour. She emphasized dependence on God.

"A successful life-changing program is more than following a food plan, so much more. It is a relationship with God." She said that my new life would start with self-control around my food, then God would use that experience to give me courage, strength and confidence to apply the 12-step principles in *all* my affairs. It was yet another awakening; addiction recovery is a lifestyle change beyond getting thin. The 12-Step program is the map to lasting recovery.

"If you want what I have, do what I do." The rule still applied. "Quiet time is the most important time of the day." She told me to pray and meditate for thirty minutes in the morning. "It is the most important thing." She continued to explain that her program was modeled from *Alcoholics Anonymous*. "They work a life or death program. Alcohol is not an option for a recovering alcoholic, just like eating sugar and flour is not an option for a recovering food addict."

She told me that the Big Book is the resource for addiction recovery. It is tried and true. "Read it each day, one page at a time, starting with The Doctor's Opinion. Then I want you to read page 449, the page on acceptance, and page 83, the promises of the program."

> We are going to know a new freedom and a new happiness. We will not regret the past nor wish to shut the door on it. (*Alcoholics Anonymous*, Third Edition, page 83)

She mentioned matter-of-factly that it might seem like a lot of work, but we need to put as much into our recovery as we put into our overeating. I must have looked dumbfounded, wide-eyed and opened-mouthed. Was it fear of failure or fear of success? I had a Big Book, but had never read it from cover to cover, only bits and pieces now and then, usually to help me to understand Carl's problem.

She asked if I was still willing. "Do you want to rise above your addiction once and for all?" I nodded sheepishly making every attempt to hold back my tears and whimpered, "For one day at a time, right?" Her whole face smiled. She sweetly touched my hand. "Yes, dear, it is just one day at a time. Sometimes it's one hour, one minute, one second at a time." My oppression lifted. Hope flowed into my veins.

She continued to give me my instructions. "I want you to read the daily meditation from the *Twenty-Four Hours a Day* Book published by Hazelden. People call it 'the little black book.'" She told me to thank God for yesterday, ask Him for help today, and paraphrase the first three steps in simple terms, "I am powerless over food, people, places and things. God can help me. I will let Him by turning my will and my life over to His care today." Then I was told to memorize the third-step prayer. "Say it whenever you feel like overeating. Learn one line at a time until it is an automatic response to a food thought.

> God, I offer myself to Thee—to build with me and do with me as Thou wilt. Relieve me of the bondage of self, that I may better do Thy will. Take away my difficulties, that victory over them may bear witness to those I would help of Thy power, Thy love, and Thy Way of Life. May I do Thy will always! (*Alcoholics Anonymous*, Third Edition, page 63)

Her final words encouraged me the most, "I'll pray for you, and you pray for me." This was a new ball game, so to speak. I was ready to hit a home run. On July 23, 1988, new life started to emerge. I had more than hope. I was learning skills to succeed one day at a time. I envisioned a caterpillar growing inside his cocoon. One day it would fly away as a beautiful butterfly, free at last.

Dawn's Early Light

The alarm rang. It was 6 A.M., my first day of abstinence. I fell to my knees and prayed for the willingness to see and do God's will. I gathered my books and read my page of the Big Book, The Doctor's Opinion. I was awestruck. My mind and heart saw the doctor's words cleverly confirming my personal revelations. For me as a food addict, excess food, sugar and flour are just like alcohol is to the alcoholic.

> The only relief we have to suggest is entire abstinence. (*Alcoholics Anonymous*, Third Edition, page xxviii)

Okay, Lord, I get it. I am not weird or crazy. I have a disease. I have a sickness. I need my medicine. I need to abstain from sugar, flour, and excessive quantities. I also need to depend on You, Lord, for help. I know this is the truth. There is no other way for me. I tried it all. This is the end of the line. The choice is life or death. I choose life.

My friends and family members continued to coerce me into believing a little self-control was my cure. Acceptance of myself as a food addict with all its peculiarities, was necessary. People do not need to understand the intricacies of the addicted body and mind, but the addict needs a sure foundation of the truth. Namely, we are different from the normal eater. It is okay. We have a disease.

> ...The delusion that we are like other people, or presently may be, has to be smashed... (*Alcoholics Anonymous*, Third Edition, page 30)

I made a commitment to do an in-depth study of the Twelve Steps with a group of serious, abstinent people, and I continued to read the Big Book to gain more understanding about the cunning and baffling aspects of addiction. I directed my attention to *my* attitudes, *my* responses, and *my* responsibilities. I stopped blaming people, places, and things for my trials and tribulations. I found strength and wisdom in understanding God's will for my life.

> Rarely have we seen a person fail who has
> thoroughly followed our path. Those who do
> not recover are people who cannot or will not
> completely give themselves to this simple
> program... (*Alcoholics Anonymous*, Third
> Edition, page 58)

Progress, Not Perfection

I stood at the threshold of my new life. My impression of the steps was basic, but powerful. God opened my eyes to dig deeper as I got stronger.

Step 1: We admitted we were powerless over our food addiction—that our lives had become unmanageable.

I admitted that I was out of control. No matter how hard I tried, I could not stop overeating. In 12-step halls, I heard, "self-will run riot." My overeating was destroying my health and my relationships with family, friends, and even God. I was spiraling downhill fast. My life was falling apart.

Step 2: Came to believe that a power greater than ourselves could restore us to sanity.

I believed in God's love and His ability to restore me, but I needed to learn new coping skills. Therefore, the "power greater than myself" was the group of people who were living free from food obsession and overeating one day a time. I was hopeful. What God did for them, He could do for me.

Step 3: Made a decision to turn o1ur will and our lives over to the care of God as we understood Him.

I gave up. "Let go and let God" is the slogan that goes hand-in-hand with this step. I let go of my old way of doing things, and I started listening, learning and living in the solution (i.e., I became a dedicated and committed 12-stepper.) Practicing the tools became an integral part of my life. Meetings, phone calls, literature—especially reading the Big Book, committing my food plan to a sponsor, love and service, anonymity, writing were all instrumental in my forward surge. When I turned my will and my life over to God, my whole world changed—physically, emotionally and spiritually.

Step 4: Made a searching and fearless moral inventory of ourselves.

Initially, the fifteen questions from the newcomer's kit revealed my sorry state of affairs. When I committed to 12-step work, I kept my secrets, thoughts, and feelings in a daily journal.

Step 5: Admitted to God, to ourselves, and to another human being the exact nature of our wrongs.

God and I knew that I had problems. That was easy. The hard part was admitting to another person that I had a warped relationship with food. I talked to my cousin and my friend, which was a beginning. In program, I talked to friends at meetings and on the telephone, and I talked to my new sponsor. I soon learned that I was not alone.

Step 6: Were entirely ready to have God remove all these defects of character.

In Step Six, the head connects to the heart. My head had to be convinced that my heart knew best. I wanted to follow God (my heart), but my self-control and defiant nature were deeply rooted in my dysfunctional lifestyle (my head).

Step 7: Humbly asked Him to remove our shortcomings.

I became willing to say, "I can't, You can. Please help me, God."

Step 8: Made a list of all persons we had harmed and became willing to make amends to them all.

My husband and my boys were first on my list, plus myself. Yes, there were others, but I couldn't see beyond my immediate family until I cleaned up my side of the street at home.

Step 9: Made direct amends to such people wherever possible, except when to do so would injure them or others.

I faced my fears and apologized to Carl for all the selfish, self-centered ways that I put food before his needs. Dan and Joe were young children, but I sat them down and asked their forgiveness. It was simple-stated truth at a level that they understood. The hardest person to face was myself. Acceptance that I was not perfect, and I would never be perfect this side of heaven, was an incredible revelation for me. The act of seeking forgiveness and being forgiven lightened my heart and brought me an element of peace that I had never known before.

Step 10: Continued to take personal inventory, and when we were wrong promptly admitted it.

I worked the program one day at a time. Praying for God's will, I practiced the tools to the best of my ability. At the end of each day, I got on my knees again and reviewed my day. I asked God what I needed to do in order to stay free (physically, emotionally, and spiritually). If I lost my temper, made a snide remark or acted inappropriately in some way during the day, I'd apologize. Verbal utterance was good, but amending the behavior for the future was better. My relationship with God improved each time I called on His ever-available help.

Step 11: Sought through prayer and meditation to improve our conscious contact with God *as we understood Him*, praying only for knowledge of His will for us and the power to carry that out.

Prayer is asking; meditating is listening. My conversations with God increased when I surrendered to the disease. What choice did I have? Alone I could do nothing. It didn't take long for me to realize that with God, I could do what seemed impossible. My humble prayers worked.

Step 12: Having had a spiritual awakening as the result of these steps, we tried to carry this message to food addicts, and to practice these principles in all our affairs.

I carried the torch. God blessed me with an amazing gift—freedom from compulsive overeating and food obsession. It was a miracle of sorts. Sharing my experience, strength, and hope was a privilege and a joy.

Chapter Four

Action — A Work in Progress

> Trust in the Lord with all your heart and lean
> not on your own understanding; in all your
> ways acknowledge him, and he will make your
> paths straight. (Proverbs 3:5-6, *New
> International Version*)

Baby Steps

The 12-step program, as outlined by the Big Book of
Alcoholics Anonymous, is not a "religious" but a spiritual
journey. The recovering addict is restored, rejuvenated, and
revived to physical and emotional health through trust and
confidence in a spiritual connection with "a higher
power." When we surrender, we begin the process of letting
go of our attempts to control our environment. Accepting
that there is "a higher power" is a first baby step toward
finding and knowing God.

Food addicts surrender to a food plan through the help of
recovering food addicts, humbly admitting that we tried to
stop overeating by stringent resolves to diet repeatedly, but
we failed. Each time we fell on our faces, we became more
frustrated and more desperate. When we gave up,
recovering food addicts helped us to see that we have a
physical, emotional and spiritual malady. In time, we started

61

to see God, *as we understand Him*, working in our lives.

I have witnessed awesome transformations where the light of God's glory opened the eyes of people who were blinded by hurt, anger and resentment. Slowly, little awakenings, casual thoughts, and spontaneous realizations touch the hearts of skeptics. As they remain abstinent day after day, negative thinking dissipates as positive, life-giving strength flows in. They learn to "let go and let God" in everything.

> This is the how and why of it. First of all, we had to quit playing God. It didn't work. Next, we decided that hereafter in this drama of life, God was going to be our Director. He is the Principal; we are His agents. He is the Father, and we are His children. Most good ideas are simple, and this concept was the keystone of the new and triumphant arch through which we pass to freedom. (*Alcoholics Anonymous*, Third Edition, page 62)

First Things First

Grocery list in hand, I gathered my gumption and walked into the grocery store quivering in fear because of my past experiences in places like these. History is history. How many times had I walked into a marketplace fully intending to buy the right foods for my diet of the day? How many times did the sight of some scrumptious temptation tantalize my taste buds? In the blink of an eye and without much of a fight at all, I would choose to wait one more day and splurge one last time.

Today is different. I have a choice between life and death, and I choose life! Please, God, help me buy only the food I need today. I can't do this alone. Give me the strength and willingness to ignore the aisles of junk food. I need to focus my attention on this new diet, oh, I mean "food plan." I am not on a diet anymore. This is a way of life, a lifestyle change.

Oat bran, oatmeal and rice... my grocery list began. Easily enough, I found the boxes and bags without a hitch. Lots of vegetables and some fruits... I marched to the fresh produce department. My mouth began salivating when I spied the delectable rosy red apples. Carefully inspecting the biggest, most beautiful ones, I placed my exquisite find in a plastic bag and cradled it in the palm of my hand. *If I only get one apple, it's going to be luscious and grand.*

Potatoes were next on my list. I loved the robust flavor of russet potatoes. The hearty skins were chewy, and the inners were firm and solid - more money for your buck, so to speak. Dissatisfied with the raunchy selection available, I summoned the store clerk who hurried to the storeroom and brought out another pile to add to the slim pickings. I found my prize in a gorgeous, brunette beauty, probably ten or twelve ounces, no word of a lie. I then tossed some salad fixings into my carriage, grabbed some carrots and proceeded to the condiments.

Not expecting much of a response, I approached the little girl stocking the shelves. "Do you know where I could find a low-calorie salad dressing without sugar or artificial sweetener? She shrugged her shoulders as if to say, "I don't know and I don't care." My diet mentality wanted it all, no calories, no sugar, no artificial sweeteners.

I began my hunt for the perfect salad dressing. It was mission impossible. After examining label after label, I reluctantly succumbed to the truth that every low-calorie, low-fat salad dressing had one "no-no" or another. I settled for Paul Newman's Olive Oil and Vinegar. It was not low in calories, but it was free from sugar and artificial sweetener, and the proceeds were contributed to a good cause. I closed the door on that subject and moved to the next item on my list.

Plain yogurt... *sounds like swamp food to me. If I can find one with fruit and no sugar or artificial sweetener, that will be good enough.* Scouring the labels on each container, I was determined to find one that would fit the bill. No luck. Another surrender. *Plain yogurt will be fine. My sponsor said that it is only food, like gas for the tank of my car. I wonder if I'll ever feel that way.*

Only a few more things left to buy... chicken, eggs, ground beef, and tuna. It was a simple stroll down the refrigerator aisle with a slight detour to grab the tuna. Before I knew it, I was ready to check out. As I worked my way to the front of the store, I picked up a few groceries for the family.

My sponsor's words warbled in my head. ***My food is my food; everything else is not my food. It is not an option to overeat, no matter what is happening in my circumstances or how I feel.*** On purpose, I chose a check-out line free from temptations. With a bold sense of accomplishment, I paid for my food and sauntered out the door elated. *I did it...we did it. Thank you, God.* Willingness replaced my defiance. Faith replaced my fear.

Easy Does It

"Sunshine on my shoulders makes me happy." *Yes, John Denver, I concur.* With a leap in my step and joy in my heart, I jumped out of bed, put the coffee on and fell to my knees in humble adoration and gratitude. *Lord, thank you, thank you, thank you. I will be forever grateful. You have answered my prayer.* With a sly smile and a chuckle, *why did You wait so long? I know...You know what You're doing. I am stubborn, but I am listening today.*

The sun was shining, at least for me anyway. The toasty warm brilliance felt as if God had wrapped His loving arms around my entire being. Joy filled me to the brim.

It was 8 A.M., time to call my sponsor. My food plan was simple, The 301 Plan, three meals a day with nothing in between, except black coffee, tea or water, one day at a time.

Breakfast:
1 oz. Oatmeal, measured dry and cooked with ½ cup water
1 cup plain yogurt
1 fruit

Lunch:
½ cup protein
1 cup cooked vegetables
2 cups salad
1 T. regular salad dressing (no sugar or sweeteners)

Dinner:
Same as lunch with one addition—a potato or ½ cup of rice.

I poured my coffee, splashed a little milk in it, and dialed the number. *I don't think a little milk could hurt. It's not sugar or flour. Milk is okay.* It took two seconds to report my food. My heart started palpitating. Swallowing my self-sufficiency, I peeped, "Is it okay if I dribble a tad of skim milk in my coffee?" She retorted most emphatically, "The plan is three meals a day with *nothing* in between. Milk is food." The words were like daggers piercing my heart. My spine arched; my intentions hung in the air. Somberly I bid her farewell and hung up the phone.

I stared at my half-finished cup of coffee. *She is over the edge, maybe even crazy. Skim milk only has 80 calories in a whole cup.* God graciously entered the messy scene developing in my mind with His sympathetic spirit and nudged me ever so gently, "Can you do it for one day?" Still negotiating, I muttered, "Maybe."

Angrily, I opened my Big Book to Chapter Five, "How It Works." I read about surrender, needing help, and needing God. Then it came to me:

> Half measures availed us nothing. We stood at
> the turning point. We asked His protection
> and care with *complete* abandon. (*Alcoholics*

Anonymous, Third Edition, page 59)

"Okay, Lord, I will give you my milk, too, but I'm not happy about it."

Amusingly enough, my coffee tasted more enticing and better than ever. It took three gulps before I professed, "This will be okay. I like it. I can do this." I had hurdled my first obstacle, and I didn't die. I fell to my knees and said, "Thank you, God."

Bump in the Road

Our minivan was strategically packed with cooler, grill, special cooking supplies, and the usual bags and baggage. We were ready to roll. One amazing week of abstinence under my not-so-tight belt, I faced my first vacation without food. As I adjusted my seat belt, I drifted into a trance, totally engrossed in self-pity. *What am I going to do for a whole week at the beach?* Vacations were supposed to be fun. *How in the world do you have fun without food?* It was a mystery to me.

Carl and the boys loved the beach. Dan was eight and Joe was six at the time. We had vacationed near the ocean every year since before the children were born. It was tradition. With joyful anticipation, Carl engaged the boys in conversation. I faked a smile. They reminisced about their walks on the beach, the sand castles, the fishing, and the food. I contributed nothing. Vacations were all about eating in my book.

As we traveled from one town to the next, Dan and Joe munched on their packets of travel supplies. Little bags of penny candy kept them occupied and content until we reached our first milestone. "Are we at McDonald's yet, Mommy? I'm hungry." Daniel began. Carl grumbled disgustedly, "You are just like your mother, eating in wait for your next meal." My eyes rolled towards the sky and I mumbled, "Lord, help me." They had learned from the master. I desperately wished things were different. *Carl is right. The boys are just like me. God bless them.*

After a moment of pity and sadness for the boys and myself, I announced, "I can't change yesterday, but I can change today." Carl's disbelieving eyes darted in my direction as if to say, "I've heard that before." The sad truth was that I was not credible. My words had held empty promises for too many years. It didn't matter. At that moment, his nonverbal conviction hurt. Feeling perturbed, I proclaimed, "This time is different."

Poor Carl. I was a tough cookie to deal with, a pandemonium of fear and insecurity. I was up one minute and down the next. Just a simple misunderstood look would force him to run for cover. I never physically threw things or hurt anyone, but my eyes shot daggers, and my words and body language could be dismal. To say I was "temperamental" would be polite.

After Carl's hurtful glance, we sat in silence while I tried to gather my composure. *Lord, help me. I want to have a fun vacation with the family.* We pulled into the parking lot of McDonald's. My dinner was ready and waiting in my new, carefully chosen compact cooler with my hand-picked, color-coordinated plastic containers. Carl laughed when he eyed my precision custom packing job. I laughed with him. I was not insulted this time. It was comical and a tad over the edge. I had spent a good amount of time obsessing over the perfect travel gear for my new way of life. It appeased me somehow to have special equipment. My sponsor said that I needed to spend as much time in recovery as I had in the disease. This year I bought supplies instead of food. It was a big step for me to pack my meal and then actually eat it instead of the mighty appealing Big Mac.

The vacation was not fun. I walked and talked, but I actually wanted to crawl out of my skin. On every corner and every side street, I saw someone eating something. All my favorite vacation foods were dancing in the air, singing an inviting chant, "Just have one. You're on vacation. You deserve to have fun."

One minute at a time, I resisted the temptation. In moments of surrender, I stopped and felt the sunshine on my shoulders, and I thanked God. More often, I was agitated and downright angry. *Why do I have this disease?* I hoped for relief. People told me it would come in God's time. Trying to look on the bright side, I decided to approach the vacation as a challenge, an opportunity to practice my program.

The Jury is Out

"Baby, you're no fun anymore," Carl complained. Fun to us meant eating, sometimes at nice restaurants, sometimes here, there and everywhere, strolling along the beach, camping in front of the fire, a drive to get ice cream, or take-out with a movie at home. Even though my husband was not a compulsive overeater like me, he was most assuredly an eating buddy of mine.

The day arrived when he lovingly suggested that we go out to dinner. I cringed and suggested that he order take-out, pizza or Chinese food. "I'll be happy to pick it up and bring it home." Trying to encourage him to consider the advantages, I added, "You can unwind, kick off your shoes and get comfortable." My ulterior motive—I could then have my planned food. He rolled his eyes in dismay. It was as if he needed his dance partner who was nowhere to be found. We all know you can't dance alone, slow dancing anyway. He wanted his bosom buddy to come home.

In those first few months of abstinence, my poor husband was kicked aside like a worn-out shoe. My experienced counterpart was no longer needed. It took every ounce of effort for me to survive without overeating. My sponsor told me to stick to my guns, "Do not go out to dinner until you have at least three months of abstinence." I conveyed her words to Carl. He was angry. "What makes her your boss?" I was a basket case full of confusion, wanting recovery, but wondering about the cost. I prayed for my answer.

Carl tried to listen to my explanation. I was afraid that I might overeat. It was as if I were talking to a wall. Carl was not like me. Only another food addict knows the devastation and pain I feel when my disease rears its ugly head, and you never know when it will appear. Time was like insurance or money in the bank. I was hoping for a stretch of confident abstinence before I would be forced to step into the ring with my disease.

Tough as it was to defy my sponsor, I surrendered to my husband, and we set a date. The fight began: my desire for more food versus my desire for recovery, tough competitors. It was good versus evil, so to speak. My sponsor wasn't happy, but she told me what to do: "Cut the meat to the size of a deck of cards. Order a baked potato and two salads. Eat one salad as an appetizer and the other with the meal. Bring your salad dressing, or have two teaspoons oil and vinegar. Most meals come with a cooked vegetable. You can eat it *if* it was prepared without sugar or flour. Remember the bottom line is always no sugar or flour, no gravy, no sauces, no fancy vegetables, no fancy anything."

I said "okay" at the time, but when push came to shove, I changed my mind. *Lord, I'm not doing that. Abstinence is having a plan and doing the plan. I'll plan to order a meal free from sugar or flour, but I'll eat what I am served. I'll commit my plan to God. I'll be fine.* We put on our Sunday clothes, got a baby-sitter for the boys and slipped away. Our favorite restaurant had lots of variety. I ordered a prime rib, baked potato, green beans, and two salads. I ate every bite. When the waitress asked if I were done, my husband said with a snicker, "She decided not to eat the plate." Sounds funny now, but at the time I was not amused.

I felt as if I had done well. I stopped when the meal was over. I refrained from sugar and flour, and I didn't eat any of the good stuff, no bread, pasta or dessert. It was healthy, abstinent food. *This is fun. It's like the date nights we had before we were married.* Minutes went by. My stomach started to hurt. *I ate too much. If I overeat every time I go out, I'll never get thin. My sponsor always says that abstinence is the most important thing without exception. I was abstinent. I did what I planned. I'll get thin in God's time.*

"Carl, when can we go out to dinner again?" I asked as we exited the parking lot of the restaurant. "That was fun." Carl was delighted that I had enjoyed our time together. He suggested that we go every Saturday night. This began my new preoccupation, my obsession of the week. I scoured every local newspaper, the telephone book and all the local flyers looking for the perfect place for our dinner date on Saturday night. I was being a good wife spending time with my husband and making him happy. Don't you agree?

Restaurant dining became an anticipated delight. Buffets were first-rate, top-notch, the cream of the crop, so to speak. My commitment sounded good on paper: one plate of food, two plates of salad and no good stuff, no sugar or flour, no coleslaw, no marinated vegetables, no sauces or gravies, no hard cheese. I brought my salad dressing.

Each time I went out to dinner, I wanted to be reasonable. I intended to be reasonable. More times than not, I would march to the food court, heap my one plate to embarrassing proportions with lots of meat, a mound of potatoes and a pile of vegetables. Then I would get my salads. I often complained about "the dinky salad plates." Pieces of my salads would topple off the overloaded heaps. My husband once commented, "You know, Baby, you can go to the buffet line as many times as you want. You don't have to stack all the food on one plate." My piercing eye shot him dead. I wanted to yell, "SHUT UP!" Guilt-ridden, I kept silent. I was feeding the disease by overeating and justifying it. *I deserved to have a good time with my husband. Abstinence is planning what you do and doing what you plan. I was abstinent. Right, Lord?*

Mama Mia

"Another meeting? This is ridiculous. Saturday, Tuesday, and now Thursday!?! Don't those cronies know you have a life?" Carl's angry dismay washed over me. I cowered for a second, shrugged my shoulders, and I looked to the sky with a "please help me" plea. Sucking in my breath, I sighed one of those long, exasperating moans. I picked myself up and continued telling him what he could do for the boys while I attended my meeting. "There is popcorn for the boys, and their pajamas are on the bench. If you want, I'll put them to bed when I get home."

"Mama, please don't go. *I need you* to help me with my homework," Dan begged as he dragged his book bag into the room, heavy from the amount of work he needed to accomplish.

"Mama, I don't feel good." My poor sad little one climbed on my lap and held me hostage for a minute.

Surprised and disappointed, the family heard, "I'm sorry guys, but I have to go. I love you." I walked out the door. As I looked back, Dan and Joe's faces were glued to the window. Somberly their dejected little expressions cried out, "How could you leave us?" I suspect they wondered what had happened to their mother. I blew them a kiss from the car and burst into tears. By the time I reached the end of our street, I was sobbing uncontrollably. I parked on the side of the road and let God calm me for a spell. I was still whimpering as I walked into my third meeting of the week.

First things have to come first: program, then family, then job. Abstinence is the most important thing without exception. Acceptance is the answer to all my problems

71

today. Please, Lord, help me.

Life as I had known it was over. My lifelong ideas and concepts had been turned upside down. Placing myself and my needs before my family was beyond reason. *My children have always come first, and they always will.* Learning that I was not neglecting them by taking care of myself took time and lots of practice. It was not selfish and self-centered, as I had once thought.

Balancing Act

"Professional caretaker," that's me in a nutshell. Not only was taking care of people my paid job as a daycare provider for children, but it was also my passion and my heart's desire. I still love to love people, but now I do it in a balanced, constructive way with clear motives. For years, my goals were limited to being the best wife, mother and daycare provider in the whole wide world, whatever the personal cost.

Dan and Joe were the loves of my life. I would spend hour after hour researching how to be the best parent possible. Determined to shower them with motherly affection, I coddled them beyond their needs. In retrospect, it was my attempt to protect them. I wished I could have placed them in a giant bubble where they could ride through life sheltered from the trials and tribulations of the world.

My job as wife held a close second in the line of priorities. Carl needed me. He was doing well in his new job. That was his identity. Mine was to take care of him. I felt that it was my responsibility to take care of our home, clean, cook and handle all the needs of the children. How could I go to a meeting and still do my job?

Even though it was tough, I tried hard and was willing to practice. It was progress, not perfection. My sponsor implied I was soft. She said that I had a warped perception of family responsibilities and an overdeveloped sense of responsibility. She said I needed to let go and ask for help. "Carl is a big boy and the father of your children. He can handle a couple of hours at home alone with the boys. They are seven and nine, certainly not babies." She was right, but so was I. Sometimes my family needed me more than I needed a meeting. Other times I needed a meeting more than my family needed me. When I felt like I was deserting the ship, I trusted God to protect, nurture, and love my family.

Ruffled Feathers

It was 7:03 A.M. Tossing and turning in my rumpled bed, I could hear the clock ticking like a steady drip of water tapping on a tin roof, tick, tick, tick. *What am I going to say to my sponsor today? She will be miffed. I told her I was going to the meeting last night, and then I didn't go. I'm in big trouble. I need to think of a good story, if I call her at all. The truth is the truth. I had every intention of going to the meeting, but Carl came home exhausted after working a tedious twelve-hour shift, and poor Joe was sick again, wheezing up a storm. Asthma is scary. I stayed home to monitor his breathing. Thank God we didn't end up at the hospital again. Lord, was I wrong? I didn't overeat, although a bagel or a doughnut would hit the spot right now. I know that that would be dumb. No way am I going back to that life. Please, Lord, what should I do? I rolled out of bed and dropped to my knees.*

Instinctively, I heard:

> Give all your worries and cares to God, for he cares about what happens to you. Be careful! Watch out for attacks from the Devil, your great enemy. He prowls around like a roaring lion, looking for some victim to devour. Take a firm stand against him, and be strong in your faith... (1 Peter 5:7-9, *New Living Translation*)

God, I know You were with me last night. I made the

right decision to stay home. Whatever my sponsor thinks or feels about me is none of my business. God bless her. I picked up the phone and quickly dialed the number.

I was tempted to say, "I'm out of here, no woman is going to tell me that I should have gone to a meeting when my child is sick." Instead, I bit my tongue and tactfully explained my circumstances for another day. Yes, my sponsor felt I could have left Joe with Carl. It was okay. I had done the right thing. As she complained, I mumbled under my breath, "Oh well. God bless her." When she stopped talking, I told her what I was planning to eat for the day.

I learned that sponsors were perfectly imperfect people. Sponsors can only share up to the level of their experience. They are not professionals; they are volunteers *trying* to help another food addict get well. I have seen and tried to work with different types of sponsors in the program, from the rigid drill sergeants appearing insensitive, judgmental, and controlling, to the laid-back insecure ones who are tossed and turned by the wind. They want to help, but don't have the skills or knowledge to succeed, and even less ability to help someone else.

Sometimes it is a real blind-leading-the-blind scenario. It is rare to find successful middle ground, but it is possible. Through trial, error, and perseverance, we find the answers to our personal quest: What do I need to do to stop overeating one day at a time?

Queen of Hearts

My sponsor was an older woman with grown children. She could not relate to the demands and obligations of a young wife, mother, and daycare provider. Her answer to any problem was "Go to more meetings." My life was full, and for me, going to three meetings a week was nearly an impossible mission. When I skipped a meeting, regardless of the reason, I got the third degree. The gun barrel pointed to my head, she would say, "Why didn't you go?" If she disagreed with my decision, the lecture would follow; you know those talks where you hold the phone away from your ear, hand on your hip, waiting for the last line? I was her captive. When she finally stopped talking, I would hang up the phone feeling spanked like a disobedient child.

I soon realized that my sponsor acted like I did with my children. She was like an overprotective mother. She tried to control me just as I tried to control my children. I remember one day in particular. My Dan was only eight years old. It was one of those cold winter months in New England. Glistening snow gracefully danced in the air. The radio stationed announced, "Temperatures dropping to the teens today, snow on the way." Dan was getting ready for school. Our usual debate began. "Mom, I don't need my winter coat today." Calmly I began, "Please, Dan, it's going to be cold today." Back and forth we went, our voices escalating with each sentence. After a tad of bickering, I took his face in my hand, as I often did when I was frustrated and wanted his full attention. I squeezed his cheeks together, pointed his face in the direction of my words, and said without question, "You need your jacket today. Put it on."

When school was over, he hopped off the bus anxious to tell me about his day. Happily bounding into the house, he met my insensitive glare. Loudly I bellowed, "I told you to wear your coat! What is wrong with you?" He stopped in his tracks. His little puppy-dog eyes glazed over instantly. Jolted by rejection and disappointment, he gasped. Meekly, he uttered, "But, Mom, I wasn't cold." *What did that have to do with it? Was I being unreasonable or do good children obey their parents?*

If Dan were cold, he had a jacket to warm him. My responsibility as his mother was to supply the coat, teach him to take care of himself, and let God do the rest. My job as a person committed to recovery is to listen to program

75

guidance, ask God for help, and then make self-nurturing decisions according to the situation at hand. I wished my sponsor would make suggestions in kind, loving, and respectful ways, but it was not her style.

Drawing the line between reasonable love and care for the family and my own needs of support and encouragement was difficult. It was trial and error. Some days I would stay home instead of going to a meeting. It was a wrong choice. I didn't slide into overeating, but the ground was slippery. It was only by the grace of God that I was able to sit on my hands or pull the sheets over my head some days to avoid incredible temptations. Through my own experiences, I became more aware of my emotional triggers, and it was easier to accept my misconstrued motives. I didn't always agree with my sponsor's advice, but I listened and I grew stronger as each day passed.

Brokenhearted
"DANIEL, WHAT ARE YOU DOING?" I yelled at the top of my lungs. My poor Daniel looked petrified. It was the umpteenth time that I had raised my voice that day. *Why was I so angry?* Disappointed and confused, I collapsed on the couch sobbing. I wanted to crawl up into a ball and die. *What is wrong with me? Why am I so cruel?* True, he had made a mess in the kitchen. However, it was certainly not a punishable offense, nor were the other incidents cause for great alarm. Trying to practice my program, I apologized once again. It was embarrassing to say the same thing over and over again, but I did it anyway. "I'm sorry that I yelled at you. I will try to say what I mean, but not say it mean."

Dan wrapped his sweet little arms around my neck and tenderly replied, "It's okay, Mommy, I know you love me." My heart melted. I hugged him tenderly, not wanting to let him go and thanked God for my precious children.

I called my sponsor and told her my problem, "Even though I keep trying, I cannot stop yelling!" She told me to go to more meetings. "Get out of the house" was her advice. Going to another meeting was not a viable option for me, as I was already struggling with my commitment to attend three meetings a week. It was tough. Typically, I'd return to a madhouse. My husband had little patience with the boys. Almost instantaneously, as I walked through the door, I'd drink in the chaos and I'd think, "Give me something to eat." Extra food was not a choice, so I got angry and resentful instead, which caused more yelling. Discouraged, I sank into depression.

Lord, help me. I am so discouraged. I thought if I stopped overeating, I would be happy. I am not happy. What do You want me to do? I felt a quickening in my heart, "Don't give up before the miracle happens for you." A minute went by and the phone rang. One of my friends in program was gleaming. She had found a professional counselor who was helping her understand her unique challenges. "It's personal," she said, "We are not all the same. We have different backgrounds and individual struggles." I followed her lead, called the number, and set up my first appointment.

Help is on the Way

My calendar was marked in red, Thursday at 5:00 P.M. In preparation for our first session, the counselor suggested writing in a journal "to see if a pattern emerged." I bought a notebook and started scribbling some thoughts each day. Finally, it was time for my first appointment. Pacing in the waiting room, my anxiety rose. I stared at the hands on the clock above the door as the moments rolled by.

When the receptionist finally called my name, I was "armed and dangerous." I barreled through the door firing my first question as we found our seats, "How many meetings should I attend?" It took a minute for him to speak. I think I knocked the wind out of him. Calmly and quietly, in his gentle and melodious voice, he began to teach me life-style remedies. "It is a personal decision. Many

77

people do well with three meetings a week in the beginning. It depends on where you are with your food. If you feel as if you are going to eat, then you need to be at a meeting. Abstinence is the most important thing. When people say, "program, family, job," they mean abstinence first, that is freedom from obsession and the action that manifests from it." His voice calmed my raging spirit. I heard every word as it drifted into the room on a wave of serenity. I marveled at his peaceful state and knew I had come to the right place.

He went on to explain how some people replace life with meetings, and it becomes the new obsession. However, he was very clear to point out that there is a transitional stage, where an addict learns how to live. "An addict needs to learn how to live without turning to his or her drug of choice." Going to meetings, working the steps, listening to other people who are like-minded are all tools to fix sick thinking. I remember his words even today, "Why don't you become an example of a food addict who learns how to live outside the meetings?" "Okay," I said with my determined spirit. "That will be my goal."

My psychologist understood addictions and encouraged me to continue my 12-step work. As I continued to attend my committed meetings each week, I could see God's hand in my life. The promises were more tangible, even for a low-bottom addict, like me.

> We will intuitively know how to handle situations which used to baffle us. We will suddenly realize that God is doing for us what we could not do for ourselves. (*Alcoholics Anonymous*, Third Edition, pages 84)

The Real Deal

"Look in the mirror and say what?" My counselor replied, "Look in the mirror and say, 'I am beautiful. I love you.'" With much prodding, I stood in front of the mirror and painfully succumbed to the idea, "I'm okay. Jesus loves me." That was the best I could do. I tried to imagine liking myself more, even loving myself, but not for today. I had invested years in believing I was fat and unattractive; therefore, I was unlovable. He gave me my instructions, "Whenever you hear yourself saying those negative words, replace them with the truth, 'I'm okay. Jesus loves me.' In time, with lots of practice, you will be saying, 'I am beautiful. I love you.' It is time to start replacing self-debasing lies with positive, life-giving truths."

"If you were to die today, what do you wish people would say about you?" Cunningly, I replied, "She was thin." Agitated, he repeated the question with emphasis. "What would you want people to say about you?" My smile left. I imagined my funeral with people milling around. After some uncomfortable silence and careful consideration, I concluded, "I would like to hear 'She was healthy and took care of herself. She was a kind and loving person. She was a wonderful wife, mother and daycare provider.'" His smile and approving nod indicated I understood the question.

He jotted my words on his pad. Searching for the truth, he said, "Do you believe you are a kind and loving person?" Embarrassed, I nodded my head. I hesitated for a second to contemplate the full picture. Then I admitted more adamantly, "Yes, my heart is kind and loving, *but* my mouth and attitude do not always reflect my compassionate spirit. I am angry and resentful, and I yell at my children much more than I'd like to admit. What is wrong with me, doctor?" He said, "Out of the heart the mind speaks. You will learn new skills. In time you will actually feel deserving of the title, *kind and loving*." Wow, huh? My broken heart felt the healing touch of hope.

He gave me an assignment, to "Write it until you believe it." *I am a kind and loving person. I am a kind and loving person. I am a kind and loving person. I am okay; Jesus*

79

loves me. I am okay; Jesus loves me. I am okay; Jesus loves me. It sounded strange and a waste of time, but I said, "Okay, I'll do it." Today, years later, I can honestly tell you, "I *am* a kind and loving person. I *am* beautiful in God's eyes and I *know* Jesus loves me."

Self-esteem rises as we acknowledge our feelings and our own dysfunctional thinking. *Feelings are not facts.* Self-confidence and God-reliance comes when self-centered lies dissolve. It was time to separate fact from fiction. My counselor asked, "Do you *react* to what you think, want or feel, or do you *respond* to the facts and what you know?" I didn't have a clue. "With God's help, you will learn to respond to the truth" he said and gave me some examples. I have listed a few that are relevant in my life.

I think I am recovered from my eating disorder (lie); *I know* recovery is contingent on working the program one day at a time (truth).

I think I am alone. No one loves me. I am unlovable (lie); *I know* I am never alone. Jesus loves me, and He has made me in His image—lovable (truth).

I want to be normal. *I want* something to eat (unhealthy thinking); *I know* I am a food addict. Excess food is not an option (truth).

I want more control around my children (unhealthy thinking); I *know* God is taking care of them, better than I ever could (truth).

I feel hungry even after a full meal (unhealthy thinking); *I know* my food plan is nutritionally well-balanced. It is enough (truth).

I feel justified to be inconsiderate. I want to yell and scream, as was my familiar way of handling feelings (unhealthy thinking); *I know* Jesus asks me to be kind and loving. It is okay to feel angry. It is not okay to lash out and hurt people in the midst of my emotional turmoil.

I need to pray for God's guidance, accept my responsibility or contribution to the situation and make amends for my actions or attitude if they are inappropriate. Sometimes I have to "God bless" my counterpart and accept that life is not always fair. When I let go of my self-centered ego and follow Jesus, I am well. I am directed, and I find peace (truth).

Stop, Drop and Roll

When my spirit wanted to explode, there were warning signs. I'd get a gnawing in my belly. The unkind words would start to bubble up in my gut, irritating my stomach on the way to my heart. The words got ready to gush out of my mouth, when I remembered my counselor's advice, "Wait until you can respond. Out of the heart the mind speaks."

To react is an automatic response that rises out of one's emotions. Hurt people hurt people. When we feel hurt, anxious, annoyed or angry, we want to retaliate. As a food addict, I hurt myself by overeating, and I hurt others by lashing out. I yelled, complained and blamed. When I stopped overeating, I recognized my dismal attitude, accepted my brokenness and tried to correct the harm I had done. Committed to recovery, I learned new life-style skills. I learned not to react, but instead to respond in kind and loving ways. Life happens to us all: the physical maladies, the angry clerk, the inconsiderate truck driver, the too-tired, sick or frustrated daycare child or the family squabble. These are all opportunities to react. *Responding in love requires the skill of self-control.*

My heart aches at times. Two examples of my growing ability to control myself come to mind. One day not long ago, being the over-protective mother that I am, I was ready to pounce on my husband for his attitude towards one of the children. Instead of attacking him with my words, I grabbed my notebook and with great vigor, wrote all the nasty things

I wanted to spit at him. Later, when I settled down, I calmly and respectfully told him my thoughts. It was fruitful. He listened. In the past, he didn't hear beyond the loudness of my voice.

Communication with children holds unique challenges. I remember one day when Dan was around twelve or thirteen. Annoyed at something I had said, he strutted angrily down the hall with his nose in the air. He slammed his bedroom door and yelled, "I hate you, Mommy!" Initially it hurt. It hurt a lot. Before program, I would have been furious. In recovery, I waited until I could respond. It wasn't long before I realized that it was just a feeling, and feelings are not facts. Responding graciously, I said, "I see that you are upset with me. Let me know when you want to talk. I love you." Allowing my children to express their feelings helped me express mine.

Stepping Up

As Chester, the curious donkey, peered into the well, he fell head-over-heels down the shaft. Gathering his strength, he struggled to his feet and wailed for help. The farmer came running, but despite many attempts to rescue the poor animal, he grew weary. No success. The neighbors were summoned, but even with all their brainstorming and best intentions, they couldn't find a way to set Chester free. In utter despair, the farmer who owned Chester, and had become quite fond of him, decided to put him out of his misery by burying him to death.

The first shovelful of dirt came piling down upon Chester's back. He felt it, shook it off, and stepped up. The second shovelful of dirt came barreling down on poor Chester's back. He felt it, shook it off and stepped up. Shovelful after shovelful was dumped on Chester's back. Each time he felt the dirt fall on him, he shook it off and stepped up. In time, he was on level ground and walked free.

I am like Chester. I have had lots of "dirt" dumped on my

back through the years, but I have learned to "shake it off" and "step up."

One Day at a Time

Over and over again I heard, "Read page 449 in the Big Book." I read it every day as a constant reminder to let go of my anger, defiance, and attempts to control everything and everybody. I needed to "let go and let God."

> Acceptance is the answer to *all* my problems today. When I am disturbed, it is because I find some person, place, thing, or situation—some fact of my life—unacceptable to me, and I can find no serenity until I accept that person, place, thing, or situation as being exactly the way it is supposed to be at this moment. (*Alcoholics Anonymous*, Third Edition, page 449)

Paul proclaims a similar message in his letter to the Philippians:

> ...I have learned how to be content (satisfied to the point where I am not disturbed or disquieted) in whatever state I am. (Philippians 4:11, *Amplified*).

Practicing the program was not always easy. It was "progress, not perfection." Serenity comes through never-ending acceptance and surrender while keeping our eyes on God with absolute dependence on *His* ability.

> God is our refuge and strength, an ever-present help in trouble. (Psalm 46:1, *New International Version*)

The first few months were disheartening, as m predisposition needed a complete overhaul. People say that it takes twenty-one days to break a habit. For me, it took eons to sever the tightly braided cords that held me captive to my compulsive and obsessive nature. One day at a time, one hour at a time, one minute at a time, I walked toward the light. Sometimes I crawled on my knees with barely enough strength to go on. It was tough, but then God never promised me a rose garden.

God helped me endure whatever temptations I faced. Some days I sat on my hands. Other days I went to bed. Talking on the telephone to other food addicts, going to a meeting, or talking to my counselor were activities that revived my spirit and renewed my strength. Talking to God in casual conversations or more intimately on my knees, I did whatever I had to do to stay abstinent. It was the most important thing without exception. My old nature withered as the seeds of my new life blossomed. It was a challenging time particularly around celebrations, holidays, and special events, as these played havoc with my peace of mind. In God's time, the fanfare eventually died, the commotion ended, and I didn't overeat one day at a time.

> Yet this I call to mind and therefore I have
> hope: Because of the Lord's great love we are
> not consumed, for his compassions never
> fail. They are new every morning....
> (Lamentations 3:21-23, *New International
> Version*)

Chapter Five

I think I can...

I can do all things through Him who strengthens me. (Philippians 4;13, *English Standard Version*)

I Think I Can...My First Baking Experience

"Happy Birthday to you...Happy Birthday to you..." Dan's fun-loving spirit and happy heart added spice to my otherwise dull day. Joe smiled contently as Dan led the way in his pre-celebration. Their shrilling voices raised the hairs on the back of my neck. Neither could carry a note, but it didn't matter. Their hearts rang out loud and clear in joyful anticipation of another gala event. Feeling blessed, I thanked God for my children.

The boys and I loved to plan parties while Carl customarily groaned. He was justified to dread any "blessed" event. It was not fun for him. For years, my perfectionism gushed waves of demands on him, "Fix everything. Help me clean the entire house." It took us weeks to prepare for company. I wanted "house beautiful," and it was literally impossible to reach my absurd expectations. Try as he might to negotiate, I had a mind set in stone. Dan was turning eight, and, like it or not, we were going to have a party. The date was set: October 10, 1988.

My sponsor told me to focus on the fun and games, the special things we could *do*. "Food is not the most important thing." She suggested buying a nice cake. She was dead set against my baking anything. She said, "Keep it very simple. Maybe even have friends and relatives bring food." I hesitantly agreed. It sounded reasonable, except for the fact that everyone expected me to have an elaborate spread. It is what I did.

I was considering my options when Daniel interrupted my train of thought. "Mommy, can you make me a chocolate cake this year?" Without a moment's hesitation, I replied, "I was just thinking about that. Maybe we'll buy your cake this year." He scowled and said, "But, Mom, you *always* bake my birthday cakes." *Uh-oh, Lord, what in the world should I do?* Before program, it was my job to bake for every occasion. Any reason to celebrate, any excuse to eat some gooey, rich, delectable dessert used to be welcomed. *I have been free from compulsive overeating since the end of July, a little over two months now. Is this an accident waiting to happen?* After some serious time on my knees, I said, "I think I can do it with God's help." *Help me, Lord! My sponsor's not going to like this.*

I swallowed my fear and prepared myself for the demeaning attitude I usually received when I defied my sponsor's wishes. Grudgingly, I dialed her number. The second she picked up the phone, I blurted out the words in one burst of energy, "I am baking on Saturday. It's Dan's birthday. He wants a homemade cake and with God's help, I can do it." I stopped to breathe, asked God for help and continued at a slower pace. "It is not an option to lick my fingers or eat any leftover anything. No batter, no frosting, not even a crumb. It is not my food."

My sponsor groaned one of those long-winded "you'll be sorry; I can't believe what I'm hearing" moans and suggested that I might want to find another sponsor. She told me directly, "If you pick up even one lick, you will *need* to find another sponsor." In retrospect, my sponsor's doubts drove my determined nature to the far ends of the earth. "I'll show her" was a thought I held onto when fighting the rising tides of temptation. Sometimes it seems as if I was wading into too-deep waters, but God kept me afloat when I was over my head.

The big event was scheduled for Saturday afternoon. Wanting help from other people, I was the first to raise my hand at the Saturday morning meeting. Openly I shared my intentions to bake my first cake. Some gasped as if I were about to commit suicide. Others encouraged me to use some simple techniques that had worked for them. "Be sure you eat your meal first" was an overwhelming "you have to." One woman offered her help: "Call me. I'll talk you through it if you want." Someone else suggested I put a band-aid on my right index finger to remind me of God's ability to heal my brokenness.

Respecting those who had gone before me, I listened. I ate my lunch, put a band-aid on my finger and commenced to bake my first cake in program. It was awkward. I never realized how many times I had cleaned the debris off my fingers by putting them in my mouth until it was no longer an option. By the time I was done, I had accumulated a small mountain of paper towels covered with batter and frosting. That band-aid, silly as it seemed, really did work. Every time my hand came close to my mouth with a finger full of anything, I saw the band-aid and thought, "I am sick. I am a food addict. This is not my food." Chatting with God, I stayed on course.

Finally, it was time for the finishing touch. "Happy Birthday, Danny" was delicately inscribed in forest green. I stood back and admired my work. God's favor illuminated my mission. It was an awakening of sorts: A birthday cake is like an art project. I had created a masterpiece and a labor of love, no less. Considering the substance was not edible, for me anyway, it was like knitting a sweater or building a dollhouse. I was jubilant. From that moment on, I have never had a problem baking or distributing pastries at a party. My spirit soared. *Praise the Lord: "I can do everything with the help of Christ who gives me the strength I need."* (Philippians 4:13, *New Living Translation*)

Pleased as punch, I reveled in my accomplishment. Immediately I called my sponsor to proclaim the good news, "I did it and it's beautiful." My enthusiasm gushed. I was anxious to share my art project awakening, but her dead silence stunned me. I asked, "Are you there?" On the other end of the line, I was attacked by her snide interrogation, "You mean you didn't take even one lick? That's hard to believe." Temporarily deflated by her accusations, I said to myself, "There is no pleasing this woman." *Lord, You know I am telling the truth. You were there.* I "God blessed her" and shrugged my shoulders one more time.

My counselor often encouraged me by saying, "Take what you want and leave the rest. You need to go to the watering-holes that fill you." I telephoned the women from the meeting who had encouraged me earlier that day. I thanked them for their help and grabbed the opportunity to share my newfound revelation: "Baking is like creating an art project. I made a beautiful masterpiece today." They marveled at my message and considered it "food for thought" in the future. I heard many testimonies of others who gained wisdom and strength from my experience.

> Two people can accomplish more than twice as much as one; they get a better return for their labor. If one person falls, the other can reach out and help. But people who are alone when they fall are in real trouble.... Three are even better, for a triple-braided cord is not easily broken. (Ecclesiastes 4:9-12, *New Living Translation*)

As I drifted off to sleep that night, peace and joy filled my soul. The program is people helping people with dependence and trust in God's ability. *The Third Step Prayer worked again. Continue to use me, Lord Jesus, if it is Your will.*

I Think I Can...My First Halloween

"Trick or Treat? Smell my feet. Give me something good to eat." The children's jovial voices chimed in unison. Halloween was Carl's favorite holiday. He happily volunteered to chaperone the children throughout the neighborhood. My assignment was to distribute the candy to the trick-or-treaters who came to our home. The task may sound easy, but it wasn't easy for me.

Alone, with my favorite food in the whole wide world, I waited for the doorbell to ring. *It's Halloween and everyone eats candy on Halloween. Maybe I could have just one piece. I'll pick my favorite treat. I'll be fine. Just one piece won't hurt. Who would know? What difference would it make? Lord, what should I do?*

I remembered my commitment. *My food is my food and everything else is not my food.* I picked up the telephone. I was not alone. My friend on the other end of the line was contemplating her options, too. She said what I was thinking, "Maybe just one piece?" We talked about the trials and tribulations of being food addicts and wallowed in self-pity for a while. We were angry that we could not enjoy Halloween. In time, we remembered that it had been years since we actually enjoyed the food fests that accompanied the holiday, and we laughed at our crazy thinking. We both agreed that one bite is a binge for a food addict. It was not an option to overeat, even on Halloween. I hung up the telephone and thanked God for helping me fight the incredible temptations of the holiday. With renewed strength, I dialed other compulsive overeaters.

Carl, Dan, and Joe returned with their hauls. My husband was a peach; he volunteered to take full responsibility of the boys' treats. It was tough for me to let go of my need to control everything, but I knew in the pit of my being that it was the right thing to do. He distributed the candy to the boys each day, giving them one or two pieces at a time.

Out of the goodness of his heart, Carl hid the remaining goodies just in case I got tempted. For the first time in my life, I understood the expression, "Out of sight, out of mind." Wow, huh? I was surprised and impressed. God deserved the credit. I was getting better at surrendering my will and my life over to His care each day, slowly and with each baby step.

I Think I Can...My First Wedding Reception

The wedding was beautiful, a match made in heaven. On the way to the reception, I drifted off to "la-la land" and imagined being like everyone else. *If I were normal, this could be fun. I would be eating, drinking, and dancing.* Carl's nudge woke me up. He was looking for directions. I told him the exit we needed to take and then I asked, "Do you ever wish we were normal?" He rolled his eyes as if to say, "Don't ask such a stupid question," but kept silent. I thought about page 449 in the Big Book. You need to accept life on life's terms. "Acceptance is the answer to all my problems today." *Okay, I accept that I am a food addict, and Carl is an alcoholic. Carl cannot drink alcohol. I cannot overeat. Maybe we can help each other.*

I knew what to expect because I had called the restaurant and discussed my dietary restrictions as a food addict weeks before the big day. For safety's sake, I re-stated my intentions to my husband. "Carl, I can eat reasonable portions of chicken, red bliss potatoes, cooked vegetables and a dry salad. I brought my salad dressing. I know you love me and want me to be happy. I need to remember that extra food is not the answer anymore. Please do not suggest *any* other foods. This is my plan." My voice elevated with each line. *Lord, help me to stay abstinent today.* Somewhat intimidated by my spiteful spirit, he nodded his head indicating that he understood my instructions.

Carl and I had history. Over the years, my dear husband had gotten the brunt of my anger. He witnessed baffled and confused moments of utter dismay when my determined nature would dissolve midstream. Being far too proud to tell him I had blown another great plan of eating, I'd often sneak eat. He hadn't a clue. Trying to be helpful, he would say some innocent remark in hopes of supporting "the plan." The poor man would get "slapped in the face," so to speak. My nasty disposition would knock him off his feet. "Leave me alone. I'll eat what I want. *You* don't know what it's like to be a food addict."

Carl had his own cross to bear. This was his first wedding without alcohol and it was open bar. Our anxiety levels rose as we approached the magnificent resort. Carl couldn't drink, and I couldn't overeat. What a team! Almost traumatized with fearful anticipation, we agreed that a cup of coffee might be nice. The car veered off course, and we landed at the local coffee shop. We sat, almost paralyzed, and collected our thoughts.

The detour held no serious repercussions. We arrived at the reception site before the newlyweds, which was proper etiquette. Waiters and waitresses were milling around the exquisite resort offering fabulous hors d'oeuvres. Carl seemed to forget about drinking. He basked in the consumption of the culinary delights, delectable scallops wrapped in bacon, "giant jumbo, super-sized shrimp" (his words), and stuffed mushrooms. I took mine for him. It was our routine. If I couldn't eat it, I forced my share on him. This time, he didn't mind.

It seemed like hours later when the bride and groom entered the scene. They were introduced as Mr. and Mrs. for the first time. My stomach was growling. My patience was wearing thin. I was enviously watching the cordial little gatherings of family and friends. Everyone looked happy and content to mingle. *Of course, they were happy; they were stuffing themselves with all that food.*

Finally, in God's sweet time, we were invited to find our seats in the Camelot Room. The hostess told us that it was time for the meal. People munched on the fresh baked rolls still warm from the oven. Many raved over "the exquisite pecan twirls." Impatiently I waited, waited, and then waited some more. Carl could see the tension mounting. The poor man looked scared. I felt like a simmering pot of water getting ready to boil. He tried to calm me, "Relax, it will be okay." He had noticed a waitress in the distance. "They are serving the salads now." Smiling ever so slightly, I took another sip of my water.

When the waitress placed a puny plate of greens in front of me, my eyes welled up. I whispered in anguish, "This is a garnish, not a salad." Carl pushed his over to me, trying desperately to console me, and said, "Baby, you can have mine." I held back my tears and uttered indignantly, "Thank you." After what seemed like forever, the main meal was served. I sighed a "thank-you, God" and polished-off the reasonable portion of chicken, three red bliss potatoes and the four green beans that were "the cooked vegetable." I tried, with all my might, to say, "It's okay. Some meals are not ideal. You won't die." I found solace in remembering that my next meal was a normal dinner, which was prepared and waiting at home for whenever we returned. I had followed my plan to the best of my ability. The coffee was served and the dancing began.

We stepped onto the dance floor and shuffled our feet through one song. Without alcohol, Carl was not inclined to be in any spotlight. It was okay with me. I liked the shelter of his wing. We sat and watched the others and enjoyed some casual chitchat.

It was time to cut the wedding cake. It was a scrumptious-looking carrot cake with cream cheese frosting. We watched the bride and groom's lovely interchange. My mind started roaming into dreamland. *Maybe I could have a small piece. I was so "good" at lunch. Who would know?* I was in trouble. I considered my commitment to my sponsor and tried to rationalize having one piece. *My vegetables were skimpy at lunch; this cake is made with carrots. I can do this.* I took my piece. Carl looked at me. Nervously he said, "Are you bringing some cake home for the boys?" *Lord, help me.* I nodded my head and wrapped it in my napkin. *Okay, Lord, I won't eat it right now.*

I placed it ever so gently next to my purse. Relishing the thought of its indescribably delicious taste, I eyed it for the rest of the day. I brought it home and placed it on the counter. *Lord, what should I do? God's still small voice said, "Not for today."* Begrudgingly I said, "Okay, I won't eat it today." I threw it in the freezer and wondered if I would be strong enough to resist the temptation tomorrow. *Tomorrow is not here. Just for today, I have a plan.* The next day came. On my knees I asked, "Lord, should I have that cake today?" The answer was the same, "not today, tomorrow you can ask again."

All of my favorites were stashed in the freezer for "tomorrow." Candy, cookies, and special treats, peanut butter cups, chocolate chip cookies, white chocolate were all waiting in the freezer. Self-destruction lurked in the freezer. *Lord, help me. Just for today, I will follow my plan. Tomorrow I'll ask again.* In time, months later, I stopped collecting forbidden foods in the freezer. I gained a sure foundation and rejoiced in the truth that sugar and flour are poison for a food addict. I recoil from these "drugs" as one would from a hot flame, just one day at a time.

> So don't worry about tomorrow, for tomorrow will bring its own worries. Today's trouble is enough for today. (Matthew 6:34, *New Living Translation*)

I Think I Can...My First Thanksgiving
"We gather together to ask the Lord's

93

blessing." *Thanksgiving is God's blessings?* Thanksgiving is a day of food with wonderful, fancy, mouth-watering baked goods and an elaborate turkey dinner with all the trimmings, stuffing, gravy, mashed potatoes and fancy vegetable casseroles. Life, as I had known it, was over.

I committed my food to my sponsor: "turkey, vegetables without sugar or flour, mashed potatoes and salad. I'll bring my salad dressing." *What am I going to do today? I wish I could say that I was sick. I want to stay home. I hate this, no bread, no desserts, no gravy, no stuffing, no "good" stuff. Okay, Lord, I need You to do this for me today. I am sick. I have the disease of food addiction. My food is my food. Everything else is not my food, even on Thanksgiving. Help me, Lord.*

The relatives arrived. I smiled and acted as if it was great to be together for the holiday. The truth: I was miserable. I wanted to disown my food addiction. Angrily I watched like an outsider. People were sampling the new concoctions and praising the chefs for their creative contributions. The old stand-byes called my name: butterscotch pie, date nut bread, the crispy edge of the stuffing dipped in the turkey grease, all tried and true favorites for me. Drooling on the inside, I must have looked downright disheartened. My well-meaning relatives said, "Lighten up. Live a little for one day." Too many times, I heard, "Pam, you have done so well. Nobody diets on Thanksgiving. Just go back on your diet tomorrow." Quietly I murmured, "Thanks, but no thanks." I tried to be polite, but I wanted to scream, "I CANNOT OVEREAT TODAY. I am sick. I have a disease. LEAVE ME ALONE." I wanted to go home. I wanted to run. I wanted to escape. I wanted to jump over some hurdle onto safe ground. *Please help me, Lord.*

In my family, for years, Thanksgiving had been a day to excuse overeating. It was tradition. In fact, my family didn't diet on any holiday: Thanksgiving, Christmas, or on any special occasion. I vowed that this year was different. I made a solemn promise to stay abstinent and with the help of God, I stayed true to my plan, but it was a very l-o-n-g day. I paced in circles, tried to do some small talk, took trips to the bathroom where I fell to my knees in quiet desperation and waited for the day to end.

Around 7 P.M., in preparation to leave, people gathered their portions of the leftovers, which was another tradition in my family. For the first time in my life, we said, "good night" and went home empty-handed with no food to enjoy for the rest of the day in the comfort of our own home, as was the usual after-the-holiday ritual. I was sad and tired. I said a half-hearted "thank you" to God, and I went to bed emotionally exhausted.

Many days, weeks, and months passed after those first few challenging events, and different days presented unique obstacles, but I stayed true to my plan. Was it easy? No way. Was it possible? With God's help, all things are possible. I learned to accept life on life's terms. When I thought about food or some person, place, thing, or situation that disturbed my peace of mind, I made a phone call. I attended a meeting or I did some form of love and service. I focused my attention on productive, helpful activities. I stopped fighting and surrendered each new day. Thy will, not mine, be done.

Chapter Six

More will be Revealed

Therefore, since we are surrounded by so great a
cloud of witnesses, let us also lay aside every weight,
and sin which clings so closely, and let us run with
endurance the race that is set before us. (Hebrews
12:1, *English Standard Version*)

Who is Your God?
"Pam, have you been sick? You look awful." My sick head
smiled at the remarks of some family members and close
friends who voiced their concerns about my too thin
body. When they gasped at my appearance, I somehow felt
successful, as if I had reached some unspeakable ideal.

One day I reluctantly asked my sponsor how much she
thought I should weigh. She told me about her guidelines:
"In order to stop the weight games, I follow the well-known
rule of thumb, which is 100 lbs. for the first five feet and add
5 pounds for each inch after that." We calculated my
targeted goal. I am five foot seven inches tall. Therefore, my
goal weight is 135 lbs. Allowing a ten-pound range, I could
weigh anywhere between 125 lbs. and 135 lbs. My doctor
agreed with this calculation, but I was doubtful. I thought
118 lbs. sounded more appealing or maybe even 110 lbs.

My sponsor told me to weigh in on the first day of each month. She said, "Focus your attention on recovery, not on the numbers you see on the scale." She added, "As you follow your food plan each new day, trust that you will maintain a thin body. Practice the slogan, 'Let go and let God.'"

Fear of falling back into my old habits of overeating or not eating enough kept me chained tightly to my witness of success, the number on the scale. That metal monster sat on my bathroom floor, and I did not ignore it. I reported my weight once a month, *but* I weighed myself more often. Sometimes I weighed-in once a week, sometimes on the first and the fifteenth of the month, but sometimes I weighed every day. The bottom line was that *the scale ruled me.* It affected my attitude about myself; when I was 128 lbs. or less, I felt successful and happy. Nothing above 128 lbs. was okay. Even though my food plan had not changed, I felt like a "bad girl." My disposition would often change from happy and optimistic to gloom and doom in the blink of an eye. Being an extremist, I imagined myself fat overnight if I didn't *do* something differently right away. In time, my program friends and my experience taught me that my weight would fluctuate. It is natural, normal, and okay.

Years into program, an eating disorder specialist told me that she threw her scale away. I looked at her in awe and said, "I could never do that." She smiled and asked, "Are you trusting God or are you controlling your weight?" I explained that it is the action of my hand that feeds me. She said, "I know if I start eating more than my body needs that the fit of my clothes will tell me to eat less food."

I have not thrown my scale away, but I have let the "boogie man" sit there, unnoticed, for months at a time. Occasionally I do check in, just to see, and it feels like the right thing for me to do at this stage in my life because I know the tricks I played in the past. I can be conniving: I avoid weighing in so I can get thinner. *If I see that I weigh less than 125 lbs., I'll have to add food.* On the other hand, I ignore the scale when my clothes are feeling snug, because I know I should eliminate some food from my plan. *If I see that I am over 135 lbs., then I'll have to cut something out and I don't want to do that.*

My conclusion: if I am not willing to change anything, it is fruitless to weigh myself. It serves only as a means to beat myself up.

Touchdown

For a while, I enjoyed parading around in the latest fashions. I wore cute little ditties bought "off the rack" in popular sizes, and I soaked in all the compliments. I felt like a movie star. Well-intentioned family and friends encouraged me to let down my guard, especially on the holidays. They would say things like, "A little treat won't hurt you," or "Now that you're thin, you certainly don't need to diet anymore." They didn't understand the disease of food addiction. It was okay. It was hard for me to accept the fact that I was done losing weight. I had a fat head and no matter how thin I got, I still envisioned myself as heavy. Even today, when I catch a glimpse of my reflection in a mirror or in a storefront window, I am surprised that the woman looking back at me is thin.

Because I continued to think thinner was better, physical fitness became my new obsession. Where, when and how to get physically fit were all I could think about. It was not for medical reasons but for sheer vanity. My thin body was pear shaped, or "bottom heavy" as it's sometimes called, and my legs were flabby. I felt that these deficits could be fixed with the right exercises. Therefore, I joined health clubs, bought exercise equipment, and dreamed of the day when I would have the perfect body.

One day I decided to seek help with getting my priorities straight. God blessed me with an insight. I heard, "Stop working on your body. Beauty is only skin deep." It was wise to incorporate exercise in my life, but it was also wise to spend time with God, and I wanted to help other people in the program. It was time to make some choices. After some *serious* consideration, I said, "Okay, Lord. What should I do?"

Walking satisfied my physical needs, and it enhanced my spirit. When I walk, I feel refreshed and alive. It is the best of both worlds. I try to walk between 5,000 and 10,000 steps a day, except for Sundays. The physical and spiritual spheres meet on the road to a better life.

When I finally succumbed to the idea that thinner is not better, I embarked on the most difficult phase of recovery, which is maintenance. It was time to share my story. "I am not only on a diet with an exercise regime. I am in a program to learn how to live."

> Physical exercise has some value, but spiritual exercise is much more important, for it promises a reward in both this life and the next. (1 Timothy 4:8, *New Living Translation*)

Denial is Not Just a River in Egypt

"Food secrets? Do I have any food secrets?" My sponsor's inquiry startled me. *Oh no, I'm in big trouble. Help me, Lord.* I was caught with my hand in the cookie jar. My conniving, defiant nature was exposed. I grabbed the dictionary, hoping for a way out. I read that a secret is something hidden or concealed. An implied truth is a secret. It is dishonest and establishes guilt by omission.

When I was overly anxious, I gave myself permission to overeat abstinent food. I would often make an excuse to eat at a wonderful restaurant. Buffets served me well. If I couldn't get my husband to take me out to dinner, I would opt for plan two. I slyly committed my food. I would say, "I'm barbecuing steak tonight with baked potatoes, 1 cup of broccoli, 2 cups of salad, 1 T. salad dressing and a fruit." I had added a fruit for dinner when I reached my goal weight. In lieu of my reasonably weighed and measured portions, I gnawed the meat off a delicious T-bone steak, which weighed at least a pound, probably more. My potato was gigantic; I would travel from market to market to find the biggest, most beautiful potato in town. Naturally, my piece of fruit was huge. After I ate one of these meals, I would say to myself, "That was not a great idea, but I was not that "bad." I only had ONE steak, ONE potato and ONE piece of fruit. My vegetables and salad were measured. If I were overeating, it would have been a lot worse. At least the meal ended."

I also played with other protein choices, "I'm cooking a Cornish hen for dinner tonight, and I'll have xyz." I intentionally refrained from committing my portion size once again. I ate the whole hen (probably 10-12 oz.), and I sucked every edible ounce of meat off those bones (including skin, fat and cartilage, no less). Only a pile of twigs (the empty bones) remained. It was a sad, unreasonable choice. I was guilty once again.

Another consistent justification/rationalization: I remember measuring my food and even though the scale said, "6.2 oz." instead of "6.0" or "4.3 oz." instead of "4.0," I decided that it was close enough, and I ate the whole portion. Nutritionally, it didn't make much of a difference, but it was still not okay. This is a program of honesty.

All these incidents, and more, were certainly occasions when I overate. Denial is not just a river in Egypt. It's the little exceptions (secrets) that pile up to cause resentments; these little secrets take a life of their own and grow, eventually becoming a reason to binge.

I had food secrets. I had many food secrets. My journal held the truth and God knew. *Lord, help me. I want to be well. My food plan is enough.* I got honest, scrupulously honest, and I confessed every indiscretion. Finally, I understood how to be abstinent. I became honest, open, and willing. I even discussed restaurants, buffets and special celebrations in detail. My sponsor and I designed a plan each day, and I did what I planned. For the first time I understood freedom. I was happy to be in recovery. It was simple, satisfying and without guilt.

> The program of action, though entirely sensible, was pretty drastic. It meant I would have to throw several lifelong conceptions out of the window. That was not easy. But the moment I made up my mind to go through with the process, I had the curious feeling that my alcoholic [addictive] condition was relieved, as in fact it proved to be. (*Alcoholics Anonymous*, Third Edition, page 42)

New Light

The sun was shining, the birds were singing, and I was ready for a brand new day. I tied my sneakers, strapped my radio to my belt and headed outside for my morning walk. I moved the dial of the radio hoping to find something to ponder during my half-hour jaunt. News, weather, sports, rap, loud music, *isn't there anything interesting out there in the world?* I continued my search and stopped in my tracks when I heard a woman's raspy voice boldly proclaim, "Jesus can heal the brokenhearted. When Jesus heals, the lame walk and the blind see!" It was Joyce Meyer, a powerful television and radio minister. Immediately, she touched the core of my being with her inspiring testimony. I heard about Jesus. Through the Word of God, her life had changed.

As soon as I walked into the house, I grabbed my Bible. I searched for the Scripture Joyce had talked about. It was Isaiah 61. She had quoted from *The Amplified Bible*, which was far different from my *King James Version*. My *King James Version* was written in words that were harder for me to understand, but the message remained clear. For easier interpretation, this reference comes from the *New Living Translation*:

The Spirit of the Sovereign Lord is upon me, because the Lord has appointed me to bring good news to the poor. He has sent me to comfort the brokenhearted and to announce that captives will be released and prisoners will be freed. He has sent me to tell those who mourn that the time of the Lord's favor has come... he will give beauty for ashes, joy instead of mourning, praise instead of despair...

They will rebuild the ancient ruins, repairing cities long ago destroyed. They will revive them, though they have been empty for many generations... Instead of shame and dishonor, you will inherit a double portion of prosperity and everlasting joy. (Isaiah 61:1-7, *New Living Translation*)

My mind's eye saw that God had "released" me and other people who were once actively addicted to food. We had been held "captive" to the disease. I saw that joy does come when we strive to rebuild our lives, and that we will be blessed more than we could have ever imagined, if we follow the teachings of Jesus.

Immediately I knew that God had bigger plans for my life. At this point in my recovery, I was relatively happy. I thought at the time that my life was as good as it could be. I was abstinent and getting better physically and emotionally through the help of the Twelve Steps. Spiritually, I was certainly dependent on God, but new light dawned this day. It was another spiritual awakening of sorts: The Big Book had been my "Bible;" it had brought me to this stage of my recovery, but God wanted more for me.

Blessed are those who hunger and thirst for righteousness, for they will be filled."
(Matthew 5:6, *New International Version*)

I became a dedicated fan of Joyce Meyer overnight. I was a baby in the Lord, but my understanding and application of

Biblical principles grew steadily as I absorbed the teaching of her program *Life in the Word* each new day.

> Open my eyes to see wonderful things in your Word. I am but a pilgrim here on earth: how I need a map—and your commands are my chart and guide. I long for your instructions more than I can tell. (Psalm 119:18-20, *The Living Bible*)

Higher Ground

When I was a child, I talked like a child, I thought like a child, I reasoned like a child. When I became a man, I put childish ways behind me. (1 Corinthians 13:11, *New International Version*)

As children, we set out to explore new territory. We unknowingly engage in dangerous activities. We climb on furniture, run when we should walk, hide in public places and the like. We test the waters and discover the boundaries of our safety zones. When a caring adult witnesses a potentially harmful situation, he or she automatically warns children of hazards and declares, "Danger! Chairs are for sitting." Or "We walk in the house." If a child falls, he learns that the adult was trying to protect him; it hurts when you fall. In time, children grow into self-nurturing, independent adults.

A sponsor is like a good parent or a personal trainer, someone who suggests certain guidelines, methods and philosophies to induce positive lifestyle changes. In the program, whining occurs from time to time, and mistakes are inevitable. People need appropriate redirection. It is all part of the process.

My sponsor's commitment to abstinence was impressive. She went to any length to stay abstinent. She was sure-footed in her understanding of the 12-step program. Although I acted like a baby when she suggested I get down off "that dangerous chair," I needed a firm hand. Beyond my immaturity, we had one major difference in opinion. She believed in a higher power, the God of her understanding, which appeared to be the group or the program in general. I had a more defined God, the God of the Bible. Frustration and confusion arose periodically. God would tell me one thing, and she would tell me another. She said, "You're a baby. After a year, you can make your own decisions."

For months, I fought the temptation to say, "I'm outta here." Feeling suffocated by her control, I often wondered if she was the right sponsor for me. Each time I got on my knees to pray about it, I heard, "Be patient. Your sponsor can teach you discipline and self-control."

> Fools think they need no advice, but the wise listen to others. (Proverbs 12:15, *New Living Translation*)

A Leap of Faith

When I succumbed to her teaching technique and acknowledged that I had changed by her persistent efforts, I thanked her. Then one day God said, "*Now* you can fly." I knew in my heart that it was time to depend on Him.

> I will instruct you and teach you in the way you should go; I will counsel you and watch over you [says the Lord.] (Psalm 32:8, *New International Version*)

My disciplines were in place, I had self-control, and I knew that abstinence was the most important thing without exception. It was not an option to overeat no matter what was happening in my circumstances or how I felt. I was ready to grow up.

One exceptionally bright and sunny day in December, I dialed my sponsor's number for the last time. Graciously, with respect and love, I shared what the Lord had said to me. It didn't matter whether she understood it or not. I was free to soar for Him now. It was an almost angelic, out-of-body experience. My feet barely touching the ground, I said to the Lord, "Here I am. I am ready to do Your will."

> But those who hope in the Lord will renew
> their strength. They will soar on wings like
> eagles; they will run and not grow weary,
> they will walk and not be faint. (Isaiah
> 40:31, *New International Version*)

The 12-step program taught me that I was not an island. Accountability is crucial to ongoing recovery. Another long-term abstinent member of the program volunteered to listen to my food each day. Enthusiastically, she said, "We can help each other." It was a different connection as my new sponsor believed in Jesus. It was easy to verbalize our opinions in kind and loving suggestions, possibilities, or helpful hints. We bounced ideas back and forth and depended on God as the ultimate authority. We were sisters in the Lord, prayer partners and best friends.

> Love is patient, love is kind. It does not envy, it
> does not boast, it is not proud. It is not rude, it
> is not self-seeking, it is not easily angered, it
> keeps no record of wrongs. Love does not
> delight in evil but rejoices with the truth. It
> always protects, always trusts, always hopes,
> always perseveres. Love never fails.... (1
> Corinthians 13:4-8, *New International
> Version*)

Sweet Tooth

My co-sponsor and I were equal partners with the same goals of physical, emotional and spiritual health. We agreed that honesty and accountability, along with listening to God's instructions were pivotal to our success.

Abstinence was our first topic of conversation. She had gotten her food plan from a treatment center years before our encounter. Up to this point, I was eating the standard food plan, three meals a day with nothing in between, except black coffee, tea or water. We compared the two plans. My protein portions at lunch and dinner were 4 oz. (or ½ cup). She had 3 oz. (or 1/3 cup), and at lunch she had a grain instead of a fruit. I groaned for a minute until she said, "I eat a snack before bed." I smiled. It was breakfast again and time for another oatmeal, yogurt and fruit. She said, "It is a metabolic adjustment." That sounded inviting to me and well-balanced nutritionally.

She continued, "I measure my food on a digital scale. My plastic cups were warped from my stuffing every last morsel into them." I could relate to that. I would squish down the food. When I took my hand off the top, the food would bounce back. It was my food, but I occasionally wondered if it was really honest. *Did other people push the limits like me?* I bought a digital scale and started my new food plan the next day.

Breakfast:
1 oz. oatmeal (measured dry, then cooked with ½ cup water)
8 oz. plain yogurt
Fruit

Lunch:
3 oz. protein
6 oz. cooked vegetables
8 oz. salad
1 T. salad dressing (no sugar, full fat)
1 grain (one potato or 4 oz rice)

Dinner:
Lunch again

Metabolic:
Breakfast again

As we exchanged our bottom lines of abstinence, she said, "I don't eat sugar, flour or caffeine." I took a deep breath and groaned, "No coffee?" She told me that caffeine is another addictive drug. We discussed it rationally and concluded that we could have different bottom lines. I said, "If God leads me to stop drinking coffee, then I will stop drinking coffee."

When she confessed that she ate some artificially sweetened foods, my ears perked up. In a matter of minutes, I headed for the door. *If it worked for her, it could work for me.* I briefly checked the idea of adding artificially sweetened foods by God, but I don't remember stopping long enough to hear his response. I ran to the grocery store and bought all those yummy, artificially sweetened nonfat yogurts that I loved and diet soda by the gallons. Yahoo! I was happy, four meals a day, my caffeine hits and now artificially sweetened options. Life was sweet.

Chapter Seven

Living Faith

And my God will supply every need of
yours according to his riches in glory in
Christ Jesus. (Philippians 4:19 *English
Standard Version*)

There's No Place Like Home

Time passed quickly. It seemed like days and I was
celebrating five years of abstinence. It was a miracle, a gift
from God. Participating in many in-depth studies of the
Twelve Steps, I shared my growing faith. Jesus continued to
heal my broken heart, mind, and body. At some meetings,
people frowned at my enthusiasm for God. Feeling
discouraged and persecuted, I got thirsty for more teaching
and for more like-minded people in my life. *Lord, help me to
know and do Your will.* Instinctively, I started praying for a
church home.

This was not the first time that I had investigated the
possibilities. The boys and I had visited different churches
from time to time through the years, but we never found a
place that kept our attention for very long. In my opinion,
most church services were boring. It had been my
experience that services with rote prayers and rituals from
pre-written manuscripts lacked thought and feeling. I

wanted and needed more, but didn't know what the "more" looked like because I had never found "it."

In a matter of weeks, God answered my prayer. Dan, who was fifteen at the time, had a friend whose family actively attended a non-denominational Christ-centered church in a nearby town. One day Dan was invited to attend. I think it was a bribe of some sort. His friend appeared a tad rebellious, but was obliged to go to church with his parents and a younger brother. He may have said, "Do you want to come to church with us? We can do something fun after the service." Apprehensively Dan asked, "What do you think, Mom, should I go?" I thought it was a great idea. Dan went, and I tagged along.

It was a big church. I felt lost amongst the people, but I heard the message of hope loud and clear. "Jesus is alive," sang from beam to beam. The church was a trek from our home, but I continued to attend regular services, until one treacherous midwinter day. Trying to maneuver the car on the slick snow-covered roads, I felt God say, "It is dangerous driving today. It is okay to go to church in the town where you live. I will be there, too."

> ...where two or three come together in my name, there I am with them. (Matthew 18:20, *New International Version*)

I looked up towards the sky as if God were sitting on a cloud and asked, "Where should I go?" The boys and I had already investigated most of the local churches, including the Catholic, the Congregational and the Episcopal. I suddenly remembered "the little church on the hill." I drove into the parking lot of Faith Church. I was "home" the minute I walked into the sanctuary.

It was a quaint little church with a handful of people at the time. The gospel was presented through nontraditional services, drama and special music. It was odd to me at first. There were guitars, drums and people clapping and having fun in church. In the blink of an eye, I joined the many who easily expressed their love for the Lord. I felt united in spirit and in truth, and I felt my spiritually needs were met. I was welcomed and loved. *Home at last, home at last. Thank God, I'm home at last.* My childlike faith grew rapidly as I became involved in Bible studies and various small group ministries.

My excitement overflowed into my home life. In a matter of a few short weeks, my boys were dropping in at various church functions to see for themselves what I was experiencing. Gradually God called them. I had waited and continued to pray for them each step along the way. Eventually they became active members of the church. *Praise the Lord.* My husband, on the other hand, even though he enjoyed the services and some of the outreach events, only came occasionally. As of this writing, he still has not been "called" to join us on a regular basis. I wait in continual prayer.

Rise and Shine

Make every effort to add to your faith goodness; and to goodness, knowledge; and to knowledge, self-control; and to self-control, perseverance; and to perseverance, godliness; and to godliness, brotherly kindness; and to brotherly kindness, love. For if you possess these qualities in increasing measure, they will keep you from being ineffective and unproductive in your knowledge of our Lord Jesus Christ. (2 Peter 1:5-8, *New International Version*)

Our church's basic philosophy is designed around Willow Creek Community Church, South Barrington, Illinois. People are taught the Biblical principles of living well, loving deeply and serving the Lord according to their passions and abilities. If there is a need in the church, it is essential that the people filling leadership positions were called by God to do the job. Teachers are people who are called by God to teach, not just a warm body filling a need. It is the same with every job in the church. Hostesses are people with the gift of hospitality, deacons have the gift of mercy and pastors have the gift of evangelism and shepherding.

> We have different gifts, according to the grace given us. If a man's gift is prophesying, let him use it in proportion to his faith. If it is serving, let him serve; if it is teaching, let him teach; if it is encouraging, let him encourage; if it is contributing to the needs of others, let him give generously; if it is leadership, let him govern diligently; if it is showing mercy, let him do it cheerfully. (Romans 12:6-8, *New International Version*)

The mission of my church is to edify the body of believers and glorify God. With that in mind, Pastor Doug led a teaching seminar called Networking. He hoped to fit people into their passions, not just at church, but also in every phase of life. Enthusiastically I grabbed the opportunity to find my place and my purpose.

Evaluating my heartfelt desires, as well as my unique talents and abilities, brought me to the conclusion that I was naturally endowed with faith, mercy, teaching and shepherding.

At home and in my career as a Christian daycare provider, I was "in my passion." I taught children at an early age how to trust and believe in God's awesome ability and unfailing love. My other passion was equally endearing. I longed to touch the hearts of people with addictions. I wanted to teach them about Jesus, bridging the gap between Twelve-Step programs and Christianity. *How could I teach other people with addictions about Jesus?* Praying diligently, I sought a solution. My answer came when I spotted *The Twelve Steps for Christians* by RPI at a local bookstore.

The Twelve Steps for Christians, Revised Edition is a powerful resource for merging the practical wisdom of the Twelve Steps with the spiritual truths of the Bible. This combination of recovery and spirituality offers Christians an effective way to work a traditional Twelve-Step program and name Jesus Christ as their Higher Power. (Friends in Recovery, *The Twelve Steps for Christians*, RPI Publishing, back cover)

Shortly thereafter, *The Twelve Steps for Christians* Support Group was birthed at Faith Church in Auburn, MA. It has run nonstop since 1996. I thank the Lord each time I see another soul touched by the light of God's amazing grace. God began a good work in me, and He will be faithful to complete it. (See Philippians 1:6.)

It was my first introduction to The Serenity Prayer in its entirety:

> God, grant me the serenity to accept the things I
> cannot change,
> the courage to change the things I can,
> and the wisdom to know the difference.
>
> Living one day at a time,
> enjoying one moment at a time,
> accepting hardship as a pathway to peace;
> taking, as Jesus did, this sinful world as it is,
> not as I would have it;
> trusting that You will make all things right
> if I surrender to your will;
> so that I may be reasonably happy in this life
> and supremely happy with You forever in the next.
> Amen. (by Reinhold Niebuhr)

Good to the Last Drop
The Twelve Steps for Christians Support Group addressed life's issues. There were people from all walks of life, including food addicts, alcoholics, co-dependents, adult

children of alcoholics, people working on fears, depression or whatever separated them from God. It was fruitful, and we multiplied.

One summer day, I was at a tag sale and I happened to pick up an interesting book called *The All New Free to be Thin* by Neva Coyle and Marie Chapian. It was a biblically-based study for people with food issues. Stimulated by new insights, I gathered the troops, so to speak, and led a teaching for thirteen weeks as outlined in the *Lifestyle Plan*, which was a personal journal written to accompany the textbook. Members from the church and fellow food addicts joined me in this venture. The food addicts ignored the food plan. It was a nutritionally balanced diet for a *normal* eater. The people who were looking for self-control and behavior modification followed the food plan suggested.

God blessed many people with increased understanding. Personally, I was convicted of my coffee and artificial sweetener addiction. They were my last "drugs," my last obsessions. I came to realize that I held onto them in lieu of appearing a perfectionist or extremist. *People already think my food plan is extreme and fanatically strict. Coffee and artificial sweeteners are normal foods for a dieter. I want to appear normal.* God gently assured me that I was not "normal." Lovingly I heard, "I have called you to higher ground." He asked me to lay these things at His feet. I let go of what other people thought of me and my food plan, and I listened.

I need to tell you a secret. *I loved my coffee.* It was my shot in the arm when I needed a boost. I drank it twenty-four hours a day, seven days a week, when I began my stretch of back-to-back abstinence in 1988. Through the years, though, I heard people share that caffeine was a drug to be avoided. It created unclear thinking, and it was addicting, but I chose to ignore those comments. *Lord, I love my coffee, and I have already sacrificed so much. I can keep it; right, Lord?* The answer was obvious.

Eventually I weaned down to three cups a day, then two, then one *enormous* cup. My husband often tells the story of my "soup bowl" of coffee. It was *one* cup. That was the best I could do for a very long time.

Decaffeinated coffee worked for a short span, but I soon played games to mask my denial. I wanted my caffeine hit. I would make it triple strength and let the first few splashes fall directly into my cup or I would order a large cup from the best coffee shops knowing that their decaffeinated coffee was more potent than other establishments. When I started the *Free to be Thin* program, I was resigned to one cup of decaffeinated coffee a day. I held onto it with both hands, until I read Romans, Chapter 12.

> And so, dear brothers and sisters, I plead with you to give your bodies to God. Let them be a living and holy sacrifice—the kind he will accept. When you think of what he has done for you, is this too much to ask? (Romans 12:1, *New Living Translation*)

I offered everything to God. I surrendered my coffee and at the same time, I said "good-bye" to my artificially sweetened yogurts and my occasional diet sodas. I learned to love pure, natural water and plain yogurt. I considered them treasures and close to the heart of God's natural state of creation.

> Everything is permissible—but not everything is beneficial... (1 Corinthians 10:23, *New International Version*)

Making the decision to treat food as a prescription drug, I eat only foods that nourish my body. Never have I felt so free and so alive. Willingness is a gift from heaven.

> So if the Son sets you free, you will indeed be free. (John 8:36, *New Living Translation*)

The Good Fight

All battles belong to the Lord. In biblical times, when Jehoshaphat was at war, overwhelmed by approaching armies, he cried out to God.

> Oh our God, won't you stop them? We are powerless against this mighty army that is about to attack us. We do not know what to do, but we are looking to you for help. (2 Chronicles 20:12, *New Living Translation*)

I can certainly relate. *Lord, won't you take this food addiction from me? I am powerless over all the temptations in the world. I cannot do this alone. Help me, Lord Jesus.*

> ...This is what the Lord says: Do not be afraid! Don't be discouraged by this mighty army, for the battle is not yours, but God's. Tomorrow, march out against them...you will not even need to fight. Take your positions; then stand still and watch the Lord's victory. He is with you, O people of Judah and Jerusalem [and you, O People of Full of Faith]. Do not be afraid or discouraged. Go out there tomorrow, for the Lord is with you! (2 Chronicles 20:15-17, *New Living Translation*)

I became a blessing and I was blessed. Through increased clarity, my mode of behavior stabilized. By God's amazing grace, my family life improved dramatically, my friendships flourished, and I prospered in my employment, both financially and emotionally. He used my compassionate heart and my willing spirit to talk and listen. Most often, I lived in contented abstinence, enjoying a calm dependence on God's ability, His goodness, and His unfailing love. I didn't overeat no matter what was happening in my circumstances or how I felt.

> ...I am still not all I should be, but I am focusing all my energies on this one thing: Forgetting the past and

116

looking forward to what lies ahead. I strain to reach the end of the race and receive the prize for which God, through Christ Jesus, is calling us up to heaven. (Philippians 3:13-14, *New Living Translation*)

Living Free

...I have learned to be content whatever the circumstances. I know what it is to be in need, and I know what it is to have plenty. I have learned the secret of being content in any and every situation, whether well fed or hungry, whether living in plenty or in want. I can do everything through him who gives me strength. (Philippians 4:11-13, *New International Version*)

The Christian looks *through* a problem, not *at* a problem. It was June 2001. I was happily rolling along, writing my book, telling people about Jesus, and joyfully proclaiming freedom from food obsession and compulsive overeating. It had been over twelve years since my last binge. I had e-mail loops and many people looking to me for guidance. All was well in my world until the bottom fell beneath my feet during my annual physical exam.

My doctor had ordered a bone density test as a standard procedure for a woman in her mid-forties. I razzed her, as if it was a waste of time, but she asked me to humor her and do it anyway. I was a model of good health, or so it seemed. After a minute's hesitation, hashing over the inconvenience of going to another appointment, I said, "Sure, I can do that," smugly believing the results would verify my admirable self-nurturing choices in life, plus it would supply impressive documentation for this book.

A week later, I got the shocking news, "You have osteoporosis. Your bones are frail. You only have 67% bone mass in your hip and 71% in your spine." It felt as if my heart fell to the floor with a splat. Angry with God, I yelled,

"It's not fair! How can I tell people about you, Lord, if I am not well? What in the world do you expect of me?" I was also angry with the medical profession as I had done all the precautionary things to avoid osteoporosis, even hormone replacement therapy. *It's not fair. It's not fair. It's not fair.* I stomped my feet and had my tantrum.

God's timing is impeccable. A women's ministry breakfast was the following day. I spilled my guts to close friends at church, desperate for wisdom and comfort in my dismay. A cancer survivor sympathized with my pain and invited me to a seminar featuring a Christian natural health care professional scheduled for the following weekend. Earlier I had scoffed at the need for such extreme measures. Health foods and supplements, organic vegetables and special foods were not for me. I thought they were all hogwash. My attitude held firm for years: "The medical profession and conventional nutritionists know best." This time, hope held my hand. I jumped on her bandwagon and without hesitation, I exclaimed, "Yes, I would love to go." We both laughed at my enthusiasm. It was a turnaround of extreme proportion.

After the seminar, I met with the specialist. I knew that God had set me up to hear a serious message: *dietary fats are necessary to distribute healthy nutrients throughout our bodies. Balance and moderation are necessary in all things.* Through the years, the media had encouraged reducing fats, which is wise. Extremists like me, however, went beyond what was reasonable. With the idea that less is best, I eliminated most dietary fat from my food plan. Experience is the best teacher. God got my attention with my new diagnosis of osteoporosis. I was ready to change. I increased my daily fat to a minimum of 20 grams a day.

I pray that my experience might help others avoid the potential hazard that could result because of unreasonable dietary restrictions of healthy fats in their food plans, and I trust that God will heal my body if it is His will.

> For I know the plans I have for you," says the
> Lord. "They are plans for good and not for disaster, to
> give you a future and a hope." (Jeremiah 29:11, *New
> Living Translation*)

An Attitude of Gratitude
Live and love deeply, beyond food. God wants us to
surrender our wills. He wants to use our hands, our mouths,
our passions, our determined natures, our talents, and our
gifts to glorify Him and to edify the body of believers. He
wants us to let go of our control, people pleasing, caretaking,
anxiety, worry, negativity and fear. We walk in love
while God directs our steps.

> Don't copy the behavior and customs of this world, but
> let God transform you into a new person by changing
> the way you think. Then you will know what God
> wants you to do, and you will know how good and
> pleasing and perfect his will really is. (Romans 12:2,
> *New Living Translation*)

I humbly share my experience, strength, and hope in the
Lord. Sharing the good news of His love and awesome
ability keeps me excited. I have an attitude of
gratitude. Whenever I get confounded, I ask Jesus what He
would do, and I ask for His help in doing the right thing.

I wish I could tell you it is easy. I wish I could say I am
successful 100% of the time. It is progress, not
perfection. Hope for a better tomorrow sustains me. I am
not where I want to be, but by the grace of God, I am not
where I used to be. Striving toward the goal to be more like
Jesus, I make an attempt each day to be all He wants and
expects me to be. It is comforting to know that each new day
offers another opportunity to "rise and shine." His mercies
are new every single morning. (See Lamentations 3:23.)

When I am willing to listen to God, I am empowered. Letting go of my self-centered desires, I am content while waiting for God's plans to be revealed. I am confident that God will supply *all* my needs (See Philippians 4:19). Scripture after Scripture embedded in my heart soothes my brokenness, and I see glimpses of God's kingdom. I see righteousness, peace and joy in believing (See Romans 14:17). Paul paints the picture of success. He shows us how to be happy. Do the right thing and be kind, loving and respectful to others. Stop worrying and pray with an attitude of gratitude.

> Always be full of joy in the Lord. I say it again—rejoice! Let everyone see that you are considerate in all you do. Remember, the Lord is coming soon. Don't worry about anything; instead, pray about everything. Tell God what you need, and thank him for all he has done. If you do this, you will experience God's peace, which is far more wonderful than the human mind can understand. His peace will guard your hearts and minds as you live in Christ Jesus. (Philippians 4:4-7, *New Living Translation*)

A Heart for God

> Let us fix our eyes on Jesus, the author and perfecter of our faith, who for the joy set before him endured the cross, scorning its shame, and sat down at the right hand of the throne of God. (Hebrews 12:2, *New International Version*)

God taps me on the shoulder at 4:15 A.M. I hop out of bed. Groping for my eyeglasses, I am ready for a brand-new day. On my way to the bathroom, I begin my conversations with God. *Lord, You are faithful. Your love keeps me safe and strong. Thank You for loving me through yesterday. Please, Lord, help to see and do Your will today.*

I drop to my knees. *Jesus, You are my all in all, the alpha and omega, the beginning and the end.* I reflect upon the messages of His Word embedded in the recesses of my mind. Seeking His will in my present circumstances, I am confident my answers will come. *Thank You, Lord, for Your amazing grace. You have the ability of changing what seems impossible. You are Lord, Savior, Prince of Peace, Father God. I am blessed and empowered for another day. Because of Your grace, I can be a blessing.*

> Trust in the Lord and do good. Then you will
> live safely in the land and prosper. Take
> delight in the Lord, and he will give you your
> heart's desires. Commit everything you do to
> the Lord. Trust him, and he will help
> you. (Psalm 37:3-5, *New Living Translation*)

As I concluded writing the first edition of *Sweet Surrender*, I reminisced to that summer evening so long ago when Jesus said, "Write a book. Tell people about the gifts I have given you." It was the end of July in the year 2000. I had just celebrated twelve years of abstinence. *The Twelve Steps for Christians* Support Group had recently wrapped up another step study. Like the Israelites on the way to the Promised Land, I had traveled around and around the same mountain trudging in the wilderness seeking truth amongst the lies. As God would have it, I grew steadily each time I was willing to surrender more character defects to the Lord. I surrendered control, caretaking, gossip, judgment, my Messiah complex and the like. God carried me from glory to glory, and spirit gleamed with a passive, calm delight.

Carl and I were in a peaceful place, happy and secure. The boys were well, thriving at school and at church. Life seemed better than ever. I felt as if the rough and rocky road of my past had been replaced, and I was strolling through a beautiful garden, the kind that I have seen in home and garden magazines. Awestruck with my new life in Jesus, I bowed my head in humble adoration, "How can I best serve you, Lord Jesus?"

Joe and I sat perched in front of our television set one night; it served as the monitor for our internet service back then. I pulled rank as the mother, as I often did, and retrieved my e-mail messages first. Joe didn't mind. He sat in wait for his turn to go online half-watching, half-reading some book he had picked up at the Christian bookstore where he worked. One email message hit me hard. I summoned Joe's attention, "Joe, did you read that sad story?" He shook his head as if to say, "No, it was none of my business." With mounting emotion, I told him that it was a food addict's desperate plea for help. I mumbled under my breath, "I remember those days, poor child. Lord, help her."

As I typed my response, Joe gained interest. Pouring out my heart and soul, I met the woman in her pain by sharing some awful incidences in my past that looked ghastly at the time, but turned out to be pivotal pieces in God's perfect plan. In words I cannot remember now, I envisioned God carrying me on the wings of angels. My life is God's handiwork. I am a perpetual work in progress.

> For we are God's masterpiece. He has created us anew in Christ Jesus, so that we can do the good things he planned for us long ago. (Ephesians 2:10, *New Living Translation*)

Joe turned in my direction and said admirably, "Mom, you should write a book." I laughed aloud and dismissed the idea as absurd. Later, in my quiet time, I sat in contemplation. *Maybe Joe is right. Is this Your will for me, Lord? How in God's green earth am I going to do that?* My mind started clacking like an out-of-control typewriter spitting out page after page of gobbledygook.

By mere coincidence, of course, I am smiling because there are no accidents in God's world, Joe had just bought a used laptop computer from a friend at work. In his usual supportive way, he offered to help me learn how to use it.

I chuckled for a couple of days imagining my future. It was almost inconceivable to grasp the whole concept. Joe was my sounding board. He kept my secret while I waited for the ideal time to "come out of the closet" with my "calling." It was only three days later when God told me that it was time to face the opposition. My battlefield started at home. Carl's disposition was objective and reasonable, but to me, he appeared negative, skeptical and more than doubtful. He was not an easy person to approach with "God talk."

Red Sea Faith

Now glory to God! By his mighty power at work within us, he is able to accomplish infinitely more than we would ever dare to ask or hope. (Ephesians 3:20, *New Living Translation*)

"Hampton Beach here we come." [August 2000]. Carl, Joe and I headed for another summer vacation at the beach. Nervously I waited for the courage to announce my "assignment from God." In silence, I practiced my opening line, "Carl, God wants to use me..."

Carl will think it's bizarre. It is bizarre. I must be crazy. How am I going to write a book? Then, suddenly, out of the blue, my head stopped bashing God's instructions, and I heard in my spirit, "Just do it." My heart told me to be honest, open and willing to go to any lengths. *Who am I to say that God can't do this? Nothing is impossible with God. Okay, Lord, I am ready.*

With Joe in the backseat for moral support, I spouted in one quick breath, "Carl, God-asked-me-to-write-a-book." He looked at me half-smiling, half stunned. His expression said, "You have got to be kidding." Carl took a minute to process my proclamation. He presented my obvious handicap:

"Pam, because you don't read, except books about God and nutrition, you certainly don't have a diversified vocabulary. How do you expect to write a book?" More boldly than I imagined, I said, "God wouldn't ask me to do something without giving me the skills to do it." This time he laughed out loud.

Although Carl had learned not to argue with my determined will, his body language expressed serious apprehension. Unable to contain his smirk, he challenged, "Okay, what are you going to write about?" I briefly explained that I was planning to write about my life and the gifts I had received along the way. Silence followed for what seemed like an eternity.

Swallowing my insecurities, I tried to break the ice. Lightheartedly I said, "Come on; help me think of a name for the book." As we joked back and forth about possibilities, Carl's tender heart started to surface. He was rough around the edges, but soft and sweet on the inside. He reflected upon some of our milestones and then concluded, "We certainly have had our ups and downs through the years; they were like bumps in the road of life." We agreed that God's love carried us over some exceptionally rough and rocky roads. The title, *Just Another Bump in the Road,* won our votes.

We arrived at our cottage. I hurriedly unpacked my gear. Blindly I sat at the outdated laptop. Except for email, I was computer illiterate, but God used Joe's calm spirit to quietly instruct me in computer lingo. Joe had the patience of a saint. God bless him. Hours later, I finally understood enough to write and save my messages.

I typed up a storm rambling through my early life, until God said, "Stop. I want you to tell people about your changing faith. Tell them about your food addiction, your 'turnaround.'" As I waited to announce my latest "word from God," I came up with a new title, *Faith-ful (or full of food?).* By the grace of God, my life was full of faith, and no longer full of food.

Carl continued to watch and listen with an amused glimmer in his eyes. He may have thought I was in fantasyland, but he saw me happily toddling along. That was all that mattered to him. If I was happy, he was happy.

There were many "bumps in the road" along the way to finishing the first edition of Sweet Surrender. I am here to attest that every breath in this book is a gift from the Lord. Miracles happen - I am one, and this book is another. There is no way in the world I could have done this work without God's help. I am confident that God who began a good work in me will be faithful to complete it (See Philippians 1:6).

My heart and soul cries out to you, beloved friend, "Taste and see that the Lord is good; blessed is the man who takes refuge in him." (Psalm 34:8, *New International Version*)

Use my words, Lord Jesus, if it is Your will, to touch someone, somewhere, if only with a thimbleful of hope and an ounce of love. I wish I could spoon-feed every lost, lame, limping one and distraught food addict alike. It is time for me to "let go and let God." Into His hands, I place my trust, my confident expectation and my hope. God bless you and keep you safe until we meet again on earth or in heaven.

> I pray that Christ will be more and more at home in your hearts as you trust in him. May your roots go down deep into the soil of God's marvelous love. And may you have the power to understand, as all God's people should, how wide, how long, how high, and how deep his love really is. May you experience the love of Christ, though it is so great you will never fully understand it. Then you will be filled with the fullness of life and power that comes from God.

(Ephesians 3: 17-19, *New Living Translation*)

The Long and Winding Road
There is an appointed time for everything. And
there is a time for every event under
heaven... (Ecclesiastes 3:1, *New American
Standard*)

As I sat watching the movie, "Conversations with God"
with a recovering food addict/friend [August 2013], I cried
through the man's journey, but then heard God say to me,
almost audibly, "It's time." It's finally time. I waited almost
ten years to hear those words. "It's time for what, Lord?"
Time to share the good news of recovery through meetings,
an interactive blog, flyers to churches, posters in church halls
or on grocery store bulletin boards. It's time to publish your
book. (The first edition of *Sweet Surrender* was published in
November, 2013.)

Years ago, I heard over and over again "build it and they
will come." I thought God meant NOW (at that time), but I
am seeing today that I had more to learn. I needed more
experience, more strength, more hope, more faith.   I was at
the growing-mustard-seed phase of life.

For every house is built by someone, but God is
the builder of everything. (Hebrews 3:5, *New
International Version*)

I am not saying that I have arrived, not at all, but I am
ready and willing to step out and see if God parts the sea, so
to speak. He didn't part the Red Sea until Moses stepped into
it. In the same way, I won't know if this ministry will grow
unless I step out in faith and do my 1%.

"God, bless it or block it. Your will, not mine, be done."

Let us not become weary in doing good, for at

the proper time we will reap a harvest if we do
not give up. (Galatians 6:9, *New International
Version*)

Chapter Eight

Recovery—A Way of Life

Whether you turn to the right or to the left,
your ears will hear a voice behind you, saying,
"This is the way; walk in it." (Isaiah 30:21, *New
International Version*)

The First Step

Freedom from yo-yo dieting, overeating and compulsive
and/or addictive eating is the goal. A *healthy* body is an
obvious manifestation of success. However, many find other
surprising benefits when they surrender to the reality that
they suffer from the disease of food addiction. They
recognize a peace that passes all understanding and, in time,
find happiness and joy in trusting God each new day. It is a
sweet surrender.

> When the Holy Spirit controls our lives, he will
> produce this kind of fruit in us: love, joy,
> peace, patience, kindness, goodness,
> faithfulness, gentleness and self-control...
> (Galatians 5:22-23, *The Living Bible*)

The recovery solution for compulsive and/or
addictive eating is a controversial subject. There are
many opinions and many sources of information. My

129

personal experience taught me to investigate the possibilities. I asked God to help me discern the truth *for me* as a food addict. I had already tried many different approaches and different food plans in my search for relief from my obsession with food. Eventually, I got sick and tired of being sick and tired. *Sweet Surrender* is *my* testimony; *my* experience, strength and hope; *my* conclusion thus far. I humbly admit that I only know what I think I know. I can only share what God has revealed to me in my years of abstinence, and I admit that there are different strokes for different folks.

I strongly encourage everyone to consider a *healthy* plan of eating. With the help of God, it is best to consult with a physician, dietitian, or nutritionist for the best solution to an individual's dietary needs. Abstinence (recovery from yo-yo dieting, overeating and food obsession) is having a plan of eating and doing that plan, whatever it is.

The 12 steps from the Christian perspective and the outreach ministry of *Full of Faith* go beyond the physical, beyond the food plan. Emotional and spiritual healing comes with God's Word realized and activated. We can share our love and knowledge of Jesus and let go of the differences in our individual committed food plans. The Food Addiction Institute (FAI) has produced current scientific evidence that many (if not most) people struggling with food cravings found freedom when they eliminated sugar, flour and all natural or artificial sweeteners from their plans of eating. In time, other trigger foods get noted and thus eliminated.

So whether you eat or drink or whatever you do, do it all for the glory of God. (1 Corinthians 10:31, *New International Version*)

Pot of Gold

One night, I had a dream. I saw a perplexed person, with no face or size, staring into a dark tunnel. The person was holding a flashlight in one hand and a map in the other. God told me that the map is the Twelve Steps, the flashlight represents willingness, and the tunnel is God's will and His love. In order to find recovery, we walk through the tunnel, where we find God's guidance and compassion.

I picture many people looking into the tunnel but stopping in their tracks. Some say, "It's too hard" or "I'm not that bad." They may say, "Life is okay. The grass is green enough," thus accepting what I call "tolerable recovery." We have options. God gives us free will, but He also offers us gifts. On the other side of the tunnel, there are beautiful gardens beyond our imaginations!

Every time I put down a problem food or let go of another character flaw, I walk through yet another tunnel. Recovery is ongoing. Whatever the struggle, God never brings you to it without bringing you through it. I will keep my flashlight in hand and carry my map, along with my Bible, and walk until God brings me to my next tunnel. Thy will, not mine, be done.

It's Electric

What is faith? It is the confident assurance that something we want is going to happen. It is the certainty that what we hope for is waiting for us, even though we cannot see it up ahead. (Hebrews 11:1, *The Living Bible*)

Can you imagine the day when Noah started building the ark? God asked him to design and build a huge boat on dry land. Strange as it may have sounded, Noah heard the command and began the work. People thought he was crazy, but faith carried him. The mission was peculiar, but he continued. We all know how this story unfolds. God held the master plan. Noah and his family lived while the others perished in the flood.

The world is full of people voicing their opinions. The media tells us what to do, what to wear, and what to think. It is time to stand up and focus on God who is the true source of love, wisdom and power. We find peace, serenity and joy when we let go of our fears and trust God.

> Peace I leave with you; My [own] peace I now give *and* bequeath to you. Not as the world gives do I give to you. Do not let your hearts be troubled, neither let them be afraid." [Stop allowing yourselves to be agitated and disturbed; and do not permit yourselves to be fearful and intimidated and cowardly and unsettled.] (John 14:27, *Amplified Bible*)

The Serenity Prayer with Scripture

The Serenity Prayer guides us into right thinking when we struggle with the ebb and flow of life. Scripture affirmations reinforce the truth that sets us free one day at a time.

> All Scripture is inspired by God and is useful to teach us what is true and to make us realize what is wrong in our lives. It straightens us out and teaches us to do what is right. It is God's way of preparing us in every way, fully equipped for every good thing God wants us to do. (2 Timothy 4:16-17, *New Living Translation*)

God, grant me the serenity

> Don't worry about anything; instead, pray about everything. Tell God what you need, and thank him for all he has done. If you do this, you will experience God's peace, which is far more wonderful than the human mind can understand. His peace will guard your hearts and minds as you live in Christ

Jesus. (Philippians 4:6-7, *New Living Translation*)

To accept the things I cannot change,
...I have learned how to be content (satisfied to the point where I am not disturbed or disquieted) in whatever state I am. (Philippians 4:11, *Amplified Bible*)

The courage to change the things I can,
Commit everything you do to the Lord. Trust him to help you do it, and he will. (Psalm 37:5, *The Living Bible*)

And the wisdom to know the difference,
Lean on, trust in, *and* be confident in the Lord with all your heart *and* mind and do not rely on your own insight *or* understanding. In all your ways know, recognize, *and* acknowledge Him, and He will direct *and* make straight *and* plain your paths. (Proverbs 3:5-6, *Amplified Bible*)

Living one day at a time,
The steadfast love of the Lord never ceases, his mercies never come to an end. They are new every morning; great is thy faithfulness. (Lamentations 3:22-23, *Revised Standard Version*)

Enjoying one moment at a time,
This is the day that the Lord has made; let us rejoice and be glad in it. (Psalm 118:24, *New International Version*)

Accepting hardship as a pathway to peace;
God is our refuge and strength, an ever-present help in trouble. (Psalm 46:1, *New International Version*)

Taking, as Jesus did, this sinful world as it is, not as I would have it;
> We are pressed on every side by troubles, but we are not crushed and broken. We are perplexed, but we don't give up and quit. We are hunted down, but God never abandons us. We get knocked down, but we get up again and keep going. (2 Corinthians 4:8-9, *New Living Translation*)

Trusting that You will make all things right if I surrender to your will;
> We know that God causes everything to work together for the good of those who love God and are called according to his purpose for them. (Romans 8-28, *New Living Translation*)

So that I may be reasonably happy in this life
> The Lord is my strength, my shield from every danger. I trust in him with all my heart. He helps me, and my heart is filled with joy... (Psalm 28:7, *New Living Translation*)

And supremely happy with You forever in the next. Amen.
> Surely goodness and love will follow me all the days of my life, and I will dwell in the house of the Lord forever. (Psalm 23:6, *New International Version*)

> For God so greatly loved *and* dearly prized the world that He [even] gave up His only begotten (unique) Son, so that whoever believes in (trusts in, clings to, relies on) Him shall not perish (come to destruction, be lost) but have eternal (everlasting) life. (John 3:16, *Amplified Bible)*

Chapter Nine

Truth or Consequences

For some people, foods can be as addictive as
alcohol," Kay Sheppard tells us. "Gummy bears
and marshmallow chicks can be vicious killers
whose effects can lead to depression, irritability
and even suicide. The terrible truth is that for
certain individuals, refined carbohydrates can
trigger the addictive process. (Kay Sheppard,
Food Addiction: The Body Knows, Health
Communications, Inc., back cover)

Why Can't I Stop Overeating?
Food Addiction holds unique challenges. *I truly believe* that
a person seeking recovery from yo-yo dieting, overeating and
food obsession needs to learn how to nourish a healthy body
while at the same time abstaining from addictive foods. To
the food addict, sugar, flour, natural or artificial sweeteners
cause insurmountable cravings and overeating is
inevitable. As the disease progresses, physical and emotional
manifestations become increasingly apparent; excess weight,
low self-esteem and depression are common symptoms.

Kay Sheppard, M.A., licensed mental health counselor and
certified eating disorder specialist, is an internationally
known consultant, trainer, therapist and author of *Food*

135

Addiction, The Body Knows and *From the First Bite* published by Health Communications, Inc., Florida. She documents evidence that a chemical imbalance exists in the physical and psychological make-up of a food addict.

For me, the intricacies of science and medicine are informative, yet pale in comparison to my personal realization that I could not stop overeating for any significant length of time until I stopped eating refined carbohydrates. I tried. God knows I tried. Year after year, I pleaded, "God, heal me. I cannot stop overeating." Because I continued to overeat despite constant attempts to diet and persistent prayer, I thought that God was ignoring my desperate pleas. Then one day I heard, "God can move mountains; bring your shovel."

On July 23, 1988, I dug in, so to speak. I surrendered my will and my life over to the care of God, and I opened my mind and listened to people who were like me but had found a way out of their self-destructive behaviors.

> Everything is permissible—but not everything is beneficial... (1 Corinthians 10:23, *New International Version*)

Go to www.foodaddictioninstitute.org for amazing fact-finding up-to-date research on food addiction.

Heart to Heart—Are You a Food Addict Like Me?
> And you will know the truth, and the truth will set you free. (John 8:32, *New Living Translation*)

I wrote this book in hopes of helping, educating and encouraging people who have a tendency to overeat, under eat, or have a warped body image despite intelligent reasoning and a determined will to follow a healthy way of eating. Eating disorders come in many forms.

Maybe you are like me. I had more than a TENDENCY to overeat! In the last days of my overeating career, I could NOT stop overeating. I really could not, no matter how much I tried. No diet, prayer, positive thinking, or mindset could keep me away from overeating. It was a constant merry-go-round. I would constantly try and fail...try and fail...try something new and fail...try something else and fail again. It was devastating. Day after day, I cried, "Lord, what is wrong with me?" Have you ever felt that way?

If you want to live free from yo-yo dieting, overeating and food obsession, strap on your seatbelt and get ready for the ride of your life! Realization, acceptance and surrender are the first steps. Take some time when you are not rushed and write your thoughts in response to each of the following questions.

Is your eating out of control?

Despite intelligent reasoning and a determined mindset, do you eat more than you had planned?

Does one bite turn into two, three, four and more bites?

Do you eat sensibly in public, and then splurge in private?

Do you feel sorry, disappointed or frustrated when you overeat?

Do you spend too much time thinking about food and how to control it?

Do you turn to food when you feel anxious, worried or afraid?

Is your relationship with food affecting your health and the way you live your life?

Is your way of eating making you and/or others unhappy?

Do you want to get well?

If you *are* like me, following a food plan without any sugar, flour, natural or artificial sweeteners is the first step, but there is more--so much more. Food addiction is a physical, emotional and spiritual malady. I had to internalize to the core of my being the fact that food is not love. It may sound funny, but I went to food to comfort me, and the food accepted me no matter what. I had to learn that food is fuel to my body, gas for the tank. **God's love is real.** He wants my full attention. **The Bible holds the keys to a life that is rich and rewarding.** Food cannot replace God in my life!

> Blessed are those who hunger and thirst for righteousness, for they will be satisfied.
> (Matthew 5:6, *English Standard Version*)

You've Got a Friend

"Help! Somebody, please help me! I have fallen, and I can't get up." The poor chap had fallen into a pit. A doctor answers the cries with intelligent reasoning. He writes a prescription and throws it into the hole, but to no avail. The painful moans continue, "Please, God, help me! Isn't there anybody who can help me?" A pastor wanders by, scribbles a prayer on a piece of paper, and throws it into the hole. Still more groans, "Woe is me! Help me. SOMEBODY HELP ME!" A kind stranger walks by and immediately jumps into the hole. The troubled soul yells in disbelief, "Are you crazy? Now we are both stuck in this hole!" With an assuring smile, the gentleman replies, "Trust me, my friend. I've been here before. I know the way out."

Twelve-step programs create a circle of love. We find love and then pass the torch by loving others. It is a blessing and a joy to share our experience, strength and hope with those still suffering.

> Two are better than one... If one falls down, his
> friend can help him up. But pity the man who
> falls and has no one to help him up! Though
> one may be overpowered, two can defend
> themselves. A cord of three strands is not
> quickly broken. (Ecclesiastes 4:9-10, 12, *New
> International Version*)

The Little Engine that Could

"Mommy, I can't do it!" Daniel stomped out of the room
frustrated once again. He had repeatedly tried to tie his
shoes. I wanted to teach, instruct and guide him. Just like
me, he was stubborn. Demanding independence, he'd yell, "I
CAN DO IT MYSELF!" I sat and watched him tangle the
laces, twisting them, twirling them in and out, up and
down. I waited for him to ask for help. It was a long, hard
road. In time, he surrendered and let me teach him the skills
he lacked. Desire and determination were not enough.

The same theory applies to recovery from food
addiction. People want to diet. They set their minds toward
the goal of being thin and sane, but they cannot stop
overeating. When a person understands addiction and says,
"Yes, I am a food addict. I surrender," he or she needs to
learn how to arrest the disease. There are compassionate
people who have experienced success in recovering from
food addiction and overeating ready and anxious to help. It
is obvious, however, that we are unique, and people come
with different needs. With patient perseverance and open
communication, each person can grow beyond the disease
into a happy, joyful life.

Whatever their title - teachers, guides, mentors, helping
hands, sponsors - recovering food addicts with experience
and success on the path are a necessary and vital piece of the
puzzle on the road to getting well. People need other people
to shine a light in the darkness and show them the way. God

has magnificently designed a plan for each of His children. The suffering, afflicted ones can come together and find God's care and protection. We can comfort the brokenhearted, announce liberty to captives (those actively overeating), and open the eyes of the blind (Christians who are uninformed about eating disorders and food addicts lacking faith).

> ...the time of God's favor to them has come...he will give: beauty for ashes; joy instead of mourning; praise instead of heaviness. (Isaiah 61:2-3, *The Living Bible*)

Chapter Ten

The Toolbox

No discipline is enjoyable while it is
happening - it's painful! But afterward
there will be a peaceful harvest of right
living for those who are trained in this
way. (Hebrews 12:11, *New Living
Translation*)

Slow and Steady Wins the Race

One courageous day, I stepped out of my isolation and faced
my addiction. It was the first step to a changed life. I
learned about addictive behavior by listening to people in
recovery. I cried with them, rejoiced with them, and I
witnessed new life in them. Hope arose in my spirit. I was
not alone anymore.

If you want what we have, we offer helpful tools as options
to consider. They are not rules, requirements or regulations,
simply what has worked for other food addicts and
compulsive overeaters. Always pray for guidance. Be
honest, open and willing to listen. God sets the pace. Slow
and steady wins the race.

Here are the tools that keep us on the road to freedom from addictive thinking and behavior:

- **Abstinence** (following a food plan)

- **Accountability/Sponsor** (having a sponsor or accountability partner or posting on the Facebook *Full of Faith* Accountability Pages)

- **Meetings** (attending phone meetings, ZOOM video conferencing and online step studies)

- **Communication** (making phone calls, texting, posting and commenting on our Facebook groups)

- **Prayer and Meditation** (spending quality time with the Lord)

- **Literature** (reading The Bible, AA Big Book, *The Twelve Steps for Christians* and other resources about food addiction recovery.)
- **12-Step Study** (working the steps as a way-of-life.)

- **Writing** (writing your food plan, step study assignments, journaling)

- **Action Plan** (planning what you do and doing what you plan in all aspects of your life, starting with the daily disciplines, which are the tools of recovery)

- **Love and Service** (giving back what you've learned and received)

- **Anonymity** (treating everyone with confidentiality and respect)

ABSTINENCE
(following a food plan)

It is for freedom that Christ has set us
free. Stand firm, and do not let yourselves be
burdened again by the yoke of
slavery. (Galatians 5:1, *New International
Version*)

In order to live free from yo-yo dieting and
overeating, it is important to make a decision (a firm
commitment) to follow a specific, disciplined plan of
eating. In *Full of Faith*, we do not have a one-size-fits-
all food plan. Your doctor or nutritionist knows what
is best for your body, however, we have some
distinctives in this program that are non-negotiable.

We do not eat flour (this includes grain flours, nut
flours, bean flours, and vegetable flours), sugar and
other sweeteners (natural or artificial), alcohol, snack
foods (roasted nuts, popcorn, chips or processed
grains), dried fruit, and we weigh and measure our
food. We plan what we eat, and we eat what we plan.

Even though it seems harmless, an extra bite of any
food can lead us into a tizzy (even that bite, lick or
taste of abstinent food). Therefore, abstinence
includes no extra anything. This might sound
restrictive at first, but it is the path to freedom and
ends up being a sweet surrender! "No bites, licks or
tastes" is a slogan that equates to freedom and
integrity in this program.

Emotionally and spiritually, we feel that ***God and
freedom from compulsive and addictive
eating are the most important things, without
exception.*** The Bible teaches us that (1) nothing can
separate us from the love of God; (2) our ties to Him
are not contingent on what we do, but on (3) simple,

childlike faith. However, we feel separated from God the minute we say, "Yes" to some "forbidden fruit." When Eve listened to the serpent in the Garden of Eden, her relationship with God changed the moment she ate that enticing apple. It was not her food. In abstinence, (4) we can see more clearly what God wants us to do, and (5) we can enjoy the fruits of believing.

> "The Kingdom of God is not a matter of what we eat or drink, but of living a life of goodness and peace and joy in the Holy Spirit" (Romans 14:17, *New Living Translation)*

See (l) Romans 7-8, (2) Ephesians 2:8-9, (3) Luke 18:17, (4) Genesis 3:1-8, (5) Galatians 5:22-23.

Step Easy Food Plan

"Step easy" into recovery—freedom from yo-yo dieting, overeating, food obsession. Experience clarity of mind and enjoy a life of happy usefulness with the help of Jesus.

This is a basic plan of eating. The amount of food you may need to lose, gain or maintain your weight depends on your individual metabolism and activity level. If you need less, use the minimum amounts. If you need more, use the maximum amounts. Best to start low and increase the amounts as needed (see the Food Plan Exchanges list following the food plan for food choices).

Breakfast:
4-6 oz. plain non-fat yogurt or a different dairy or breakfast protein
1 egg or another breakfast protein
1 oz. oatmeal or another grain
1 small/medium sized fruit

Lunch:
3-4 oz. protein
optional: grain or fruit
6-8 oz. salad
6-8 oz. low-carbohydrate vegetables, cooked or raw
1 tablespoon olive oil or another fat exchange

Dinner:
3-4 oz. protein
4 oz. grain
6-8 oz. salad
6-8 oz. low-carbohydrate vegetables, cooked or raw
1-2 tablespoon olive oil or another fat exchange

Metabolic Adjustment:*
dairy or breakfast protein
1 small/medium fruit

*metabolic adjustment can be added to lunch or dinner or eaten in the morning, afternoon or evening.

Men: Use maximum amounts, increase the cereal grain at breakfast to 1.5 oz and increase the grain at dinner to 6 oz (or ¾ cup).

This is *not* a program of deprivation. There can be some flexibility in setting up a food plan. Depending on age, body size, activity level and metabolism, a person might need more or less food to sustain his/her energy level and to avoid physical hunger. I have listed the suggested range in choosing portion sizes.

Food Plan Exchanges
Dairy: 4-6 oz. non-fat plain yogurt, 8 oz. low-fat or skim milk, 3 oz. cottage cheese, 1 oz. hard cheese* (could substitute breakfast protein portion for dairy)

Breakfast proteins portions: 1 egg or 1/2 cup egg substitute, 2 egg whites, 3 oz. cottage cheese, 4 oz. beans, 2 oz. chicken, beef, pork, 1 oz. hard cheese*

Breakfast cereals: 1 oz. unprocessed whole-grains (measured dry, then cooked with water): oatmeal, oat bran, grits, cream of rice, cream of buckwheat, cream of barley, cream of rye *(Always check cereal labels for sugar, flour and wheat.)*

Grains: 4 oz. or 1/2 cup baked, boiled or mashed potatoes, sweet potatoes, yams, acorn squash, butternut squash or cooked green peas, beets, pumpkin, corn (or l ear corn-on-the-cob), lentils, chickpeas, lima beans, kidney beans, navy beans (or any cooked dried beans), prepared rice (brown preferred), quinoa.

Avoid flour products—even "healthy" choices like whole-grain bread and pasta, and note that most gravies, soups and sauces are thickened with flour. Therefore, these foods are considered taboo for a food addict

Lunch and dinner protein portions: 3-4 oz. chicken, turkey, fish/seafood, tuna (canned in water), haddock, cod, salmon, halibut, bass, catfish, crab meat, shrimp, lobster, scallops, beef, pork, lamb, veal, 2 eggs, 6 oz. cottage cheese, 4-6 oz. beans/legumes, tofu, 1 veggie burger, 2 oz. hard cheese*.

*Hard cheese is high in fat and is best avoided or eaten in very limited amounts until the maintenance stage of recovery.

Prepare proteins by roasting, stewing, grilling, baking or pan-frying in your allotment of olive oil or butter. Avoid deep-fried fish, seafood or chicken.

Low-carbohydrate vegetables: *12-16 oz.* (Prepared in a salad, cooked or eaten raw)*:* Alfalfa sprouts, asparagus, beans (green or wax), Bok choy, broccoli, Brussels sprouts, cabbage, carrots, cauliflower, celery, collard greens, cucumber, eggplant, green or red peppers, kale, lettuce (all varieties), mushrooms, okra, onions, radishes, spaghetti squash, spinach, Swiss chard, tomatoes, turnips, turnip greens, yellow squash (summer), zucchini (6 oz of V8 juice or tomato juice can be substituted for a serving of vegetables.)

Fats: 1 tablespoon oil (healthy oils such as olive, coconut, walnut, flax, sesame), 1 tablespoon butter, 1 tablespoon regular salad dressing (Newman's Own Olive Oil and Vinegar is a recommended choice), 1 tablespoon real mayonnaise, 1 tablespoon tahini*, 1/2 oz. *raw* nuts*, 1/2 oz. *raw* seeds* , (healthy choices such as flax, chia, kemp, sesame seeds, sunflower seeds), 2 oz. avocado, 9 olives.

*Caution: best to wait until the maintenance phase of recovery before trying raw nuts, seeds, nut butters.

Condiments: *(Acceptable addition to any meal)* 2 tablespoons mustard, 2 tablespoons sugar-free salsa per meal, vinegar (best to avoid balsamic vinegar)*

*Even though during fermentation of *balsamic vinegar* a lot of the sugar is converted to acid, balsamic vinegar contains more sugar than regular vinegar. Use with caution.

Fruits: (fresh, frozen or canned in its own juice): 4 oz. (or 1/2 cup) fruit or a small-medium sized (approx. 4-5 oz) apple, nectarine, orange, peach, pear, plum, tangerine, 4 oz (or 1/2 cup) blackberries, blueberries, cherries*, grapes*, honeydew melon, mango*, pineapple*, raspberries, strawberries, watermelon, applesauce, cantaloupe (or 1/4), grapefruit (or 1/2).

*Cherries, grapes, mango and pineapple have been known to set up cravings in some food addicts. Consider your options carefully and listen to your body when introducing these foods.

An extra note of caution when considering bananas: Bananas are high in sugar. It is best to avoid them; however, if a banana is "doctor recommended," the portion size is 2 oz. or ½.

Beverages: Wonderful, life-giving water (hot or cold) with optional wedge of lemon or lime, seltzer water, herb teas, decaffeinated black coffee or tea.

Guidelines for Food Addicts Like Me

People who are addicted to sugar, flour and natural or artificial sweeteners need to pay close attention to the little extras—the things that seem like no big deal but can make the difference between staying abstinent or succumbing to the disease one more time.

Eliminate all sugar products from your food plan: Check all food labels for hidden sugar; obviously, anything with the word "sugar" falls into this category (like brown sugar or confectioners sugar). "Syrup" too is a keyword— corn syrup, maple syrup and the like, honey, and molasses. These are the more common names of sugar additives but there are others.

Eliminate all sweeteners (natural and artificial): These may be listed as barley malt, dextrin, maltodextrin, sorbitol, stevia, xylitol, and most ingredients ending with "ose," including—but not limited to—dextrose, fructose, sucrose.

The list includes all diet drinks, mints, gum, packets added to anything, any sweetened foods, even Stevia. If you are unsure of an ingredient, check with the manufacturer or practice the rule, "if in doubt, leave it out."

Eliminate all flour products from your food plan: Check all labels for the word "flour." Anything that is ground into flour counts, even nut flour. Foods in this category include breads, pastas, all sweets, most cold cereals—the list is extensive—bagels, doughnuts, muffins and the like. Chips and crackers, even without the word "flour" in the ingredient list, are foods to avoid. Also note that flour is often used as a thickening agent in soups, sauces and gravies, and breadcrumbs are used as a binding agent in the preparation of meatloaf or meatballs. Check labels carefully.

Limit (or eliminate) caffeine: It is best to wean off coffee and tea gradually. In time, if addicted, eliminate caffeine altogether. Green tea can be a healthy choice in reasonable amounts (no more than three cups a day).

Eliminate all alcohol: Some people say that alcohol is liquid sugar with a kick. It is not an option for a food addict.

Do not eat standing: Always take the time to sit and eat your whole meal at one time (if at all possible). It is dangerous for a food addict to eat standing at the kitchen counter or to eat piece-meal, even if it is our weighed and measured food. It is much better to take a breather. Sit, relax, and enjoy the meal and the time. It is a positive self-discipline that gives us an opportunity to say, "I need to replenish my energy—physically, emotionally and spiritually." God blesses those decisions.

Pray before eating: Before I put even one iota of food in my mouth, I pray. I take a moment to say, "Thank you, God, for my abstinence. Thank you for the food on my plate," but I don't stop there. I am sure to say, "Lord, is this guilt-free?" And then I listen. *I really listen.*

Restaurant dining can be a challenge, especially when I make the decision to use the eyeball method of measuring my food. Sometimes God tells me that my portions are too big. I then have the opportunity to fix it *before* I eat the meal. I simply put the excess food on my bread plate and ask again, "Lord, is it guilt-free now?"

This is a simple program, but it's not always easy. As a food addict, I occasionally want to eat foods that are not mine (referring to anything—even sugar-free "abstinent" foods), but with the amazing love and grace of God, I practice my program one day at a time.

As with any new food plan, it is best to consult with your physician regarding your individual dietary needs. (The publisher and I disclaim responsibility for any adverse effects arising from the suggestions offered in this book.)

Keep Coming Back

My own experiences were my best teachers! It took me a very long time to understand what I needed to do each day to stay free from overeating. Every time I made a mistake, I picked myself up, asked the Lord for forgiveness, forgave myself, and picked up where I left off. I had (and still have) a destination in mind. I long to stay free from the desire to overeat, but at the very least, I want to resist the temptation to eat anything outside of my food plan no matter what I think, feel or want to do.

> My food is my food. Everything else is not my food. It is not an option to overeat no matter what is happening in my circumstances or how I feel. Period. End of food thought. Love and service keeps me dry. (my mantra)

It is like riding a horse on a new terrain. If I were depending on a horse for transportation from one place to another, I'd get on the horse in the barn. I'd travel down the terrain, but I would pay close attention to the road to make sure the horse didn't trip on a stone and fall into a ditch. Sometimes, I'd notice a rocky ride and a near accident. Other times, I'd go flying to the ground. The fall would hurt, but I would brush myself off and get right back on the horse, having learned from each occurrence. I definitely wouldn't go back to the barn and start from scratch.

Just like my adherence to my food plan, when I ate an extra bite, lick, taste or more, I recognized that I had to protect myself from some thought, feeling or situation and I learned from the experience in order that I might avoid another slip in the days to come.

ACCOUNTABILITY/SPONSORS
(having a sponsor or an accountability partner or posting on the *Full of Faith* Facebook Accountability pages)

In *Full of Faith*, we believe that God and abstinence (as described in this program) are the most important things, without exception. These two things unify us and make us members of the *Full of Faith* family.

A *Full of Faith* sponsor is a Christian in recovery who understands food addiction from personal experience and is willing to share with individuals (or as the lead of a small group) in a teaching, guiding, helping and encouraging role. He or she is sponsored, has more than 30 days of freedom from compulsively overeating, and is actively engaged in working the tools of recovery as a way of life in the *Full of Faith* program.

All sponsors and sponsees agree on a basic food plan - weighed and measured, with detailed options for exceptional circumstances (i.e., restaurant dining, illness, medical issues, food changes). And all sponsors and sponsees agree on a form of communication. Some talk every day on the phone at a set time, while others connect via email, text, or Facebook private messages each day. Committing to a specific food plan each day is paramount.

A sponsor's responsibility is to share his/her experience, strength, and hope in a kind and loving, non-judgmental, faith-filled way. A sponsee's responsibility is to write a specific food plan and commit it to the sponsor every day. If there are other agreements in place, the sponsee is held accountable. Sponsees agree to be 100% honest 100% of the time. No exceptions. We don't hold any food secrets from our sponsors no matter how insignificant the indiscretion might seem.

Beyond abstinence and accountability, a sponsor teaches a sponsee how to use the tools of recovery to support this life-changing way of life. There are many ways to do that. Some sponsors introduce the rest of the tools in a more casual approach, while others set up a disciplined outline for using every tool every day. As a general rule, though, sponsors want to be sure that their sponsees are praying, reading the Word, communicating with other food addicts, going to meetings, working the 12 steps, writing their feelings if they are hurting for some reason, giving back regularly. These are action steps of a program that works. Our program is not a diet club, but a way of life.

In the *Full of Faith* program, we also offer help and encouragement through the *Full of Faith* Accountability Facebook Group. There is a daily post entitled, "In Need of a Sponsor Group" (with a picture of a plate with a big smile in the center) for people who are new to the group or for those who are coming back and want accountability. There is an assigned leader that oversees the group each day, who acts as a temporary sponsor by making suggestions, guiding and encouraging contributors. This is a place of transition until, in time, these individuals find sponsors or join small groups.

MEETINGS
(attending phone meetings, ZOOM video conferences and online step studies)

> Where two or three come together in my name, there am I with them. (Matthew 18:20, *New International Version*)

Meetings are gatherings of two or more like-minded people who come together to share their experience, strength and hope in recovery. Fellowship with other addicts gives us an opportunity to identify our common concerns, and through shared experiences dealing with challenging situations, both practically with the food and mentally and emotionally, we learn new strategies for coping with life. We share testimonies and pray for one another. Connecting with and learning from other food addicts is an important part of the recovery process.

COMMUNICATION
(making phone calls, texting, posting and commenting on our Facebook groups)

There are many ways to communicate in the world we live in today. Personally, I prefer the telephone, but I also converse by text, by private messaging through Facebook, by email, or through one of the private *Full of Faith* Facebook groups.

PRAYER AND MEDITATION
(spending quality time with the Lord)

[Jesus said,] Ask and it will be given to you; seek and you will find; knock and the door will be opened to you. (Matthew 7:7, *New International Version*)

To stay connected to the only true source of strength, we dedicate a specific time in the day, preferably in the morning before we begin the hustle and bustle of the day, to pray and meditate. This gives us the opportunity to bring all our thoughts and concerns to the Lord. We seek His guidance and direction. Jesus sent the Holy Spirit as the: "Comforter, Counselor, Helper, Intercessor, Advocate, Strengthener, and Standby." (John 14:16, *Amplified Bible*) And He taught us how to pray:

When you pray, go away by yourself, shut the door behind you, and pray to your Father secretly. Then your Father, who knows all secrets, will reward you...your Father knows exactly what you need even before you ask him! (Matthew 6:6-8, *New Living Translation*)

LITERATURE
(reading *The Bible, Alcoholics Anonymous, The Twelve Steps for Christians* and other resources about food addiction recovery)

> Open my eyes to see wonderful things in your Word. I am but a pilgrim here on earth: how I need a map—and your commands are my chart and guide. I long for your instructions more than I can tell. (Psalm 119-18-20, *The Living Bible*)

The Bible is our ultimate source and guide. *The Life Recovery Bible* is a wonderful resource as it helps me to see how the Word relates to me as an addict through the footnotes and sidebar reflections. The Big Book, *Alcoholics Anonymous*, supplies easily identifiable keys to recovery from addictive behavior, and The Twelve Steps for Christians brings the two together. It combines the 12-step approach with biblical truth. I see it as *Christianity 101* or even *Christianity for Dummies* (said in kindness and respect for my learning disability).

We also read *Food for Thought* by Hazelden and other books and articles about food addiction recovery. Detailed information about the science of food addiction on which the *Full of Faith* program is based can be found at the Food Addiction Institute's website: www.foodaddictioninstitute.org.

TWELVE STEP STUDY
(working the steps as a way-of-life)
The central theme of the 12 steps can be found in the first

three steps. This is my personal interpretation of them:

Step One - I admitted I am powerless over food, people, places and things; my life had become unmanageable. *I am powerless over food and the things that make me feel separated from God's love and care. Makes me feel out of control.*

Step Two - Came to believe that a power greater than myself could restore me to sanity. *Jesus is waiting for me to depend entirely on Him, and I accept the fact that food addiction is a malady that affects people who are addicted to sugar, flour, natural and artificial sweeteners, plus volume. AND co-dependency is also a problem for me.*

Step Three - Made a decision to turn my will and my life over to the care of God as I understand Him. *I decided to let God help me overcome any temptations, starting with the desire to eat extra food, and eventually I admitted that I am powerless over other things, known as shortcomings, that have created havoc in my life, so that Jesus can help me take appropriate actions. I let go of my denial and trust Him.*

> Trust in the Lord with all your heart and lean not on your own understanding; in all your ways acknowledge him, and he will make your paths straight. (Proverbs 3:5-6, *New International Version*)

There are a few ways to read, study and apply the 12 steps as a way-of-life. You could attend a 12-step study online in a *Full of Faith* private Facebook group, or join a ZOOM video conference or a phone meeting with *Full of Faith* peers, or you could work through the steps one-to-one with a sponsor, therapist, minister or a trusted friend.

WRITING
(writing your food plan, step study assignments, journaling)

Recovering food addicts report their committed food plans each day to a sponsor, accountability partner or they post their food on the "In need of a Sponsor" page in the Facebook *Full of Faith* Accountability group.

Writing a 4th step inventory is part of the 12-step study process.

It is common practice to write entries in a journal during times of frustration or simply as a way to express our feelings each day.

I write "HELP ME, LORD!" letters when I am anxious, frustrated, disturbed by something or someone. When I put my thoughts and feelings on paper, it opens the lines of communication with God. Sometimes I yell, "WAKE UP, JESUS!" but I soon realize that He is always awake and available to help me through any storm.

Writing a gratitude list helps me remember God's grace.

Sometimes I write "the four G's"—what I did *good*, my *glitches*, my *goals* and my *gratitude list.*

> The Lord is my strength, my shield from every
> danger. I trust in him with all my heart. He
> helps me, and my heart is filled with joy...
> (Psalm 28:7 *New Living Translation*)

ACTION PLAN
(planning what you do and doing what you plan in all aspects of your life, starting with the daily disciplines, which are the tools of recovery)

Developing realistic guidelines and expectations for the day is an important aspect in living a peaceful, balanced life. I don't do the tools cafeteria style (taking what I want and leaving the rest). I do every tool every day. (Abstinence,

Accountability/Sponsor, Communication, Literature, 12-Step Study, Meetings, Writing, Prayer and Meditation, Anonymity, Love and Service). It is not as daunting as it sounds. Here is what my action plan looks like on a daily basis:

- I start each day in intentional prayer, and I read and reflect on God's Word before breakfast. (I don't commit to reading the Old Testament, New Testament, Proverbs and Psalms each day, like some do in a year, but I pick one each year.) (Literature, Prayer and Meditation)

- I write my food plan and commit it to my sponsor by phone, text or private message through Facebook. (Abstinence, Sponsor, Writing, Communication)

- I follow my food plan as detailed. (Abstinence)

- I talk to sponsees at committed times. (Love and Service, Communication)

- Typically, I attend at least one meeting a day where we read some form of literature. (Meetings, Literature, Communication, Love and service)

- I share at meetings, and I write and answer e-mail, text and Facebook private messages. (Communication, Love and Service, Writing, Anonymity)

- I share on the *Full of Faith* Facebook groups. (Communication, Love and Service, Writing)

- I make and answer phone calls. (Communication, Love and Service)

- After each meal, I do a tenth step inventory and complete assignments for my 12-step study. (The 12-Steps, Prayer and Meditation, Writing)

Beyond facilitating the tool box, I plan what I do and do what I plan being sure that God and abstinence are the most important things, without exception. My husband comes next in the line of priorities. In respect and consideration for him, I turn off all electronics (including my cell phone) by 8pm, and I include rest and fun in my action plan.

I typically have some special assignments on my to-do list each day, but I consider balance and moderation and don't plan more than I can realistically do in a day.

LOVE AND SERVICE
(giving back what you've learned and received)

....Love your neighbor as yourself. (Galatians 5:14, *New International Version*)

Bill Wilson, founder of Alcoholics Anonymous, told us that "love and service" kept him sober. The same theory works for all addictions. When we extend our hearts and hands to other people, we become a reflection of God's love.

We can attend meetings, make a phone call, help a newcomer get started in the program, or call a friend or family member to say, "I care about you." Maybe we can volunteer to help at a nursing home, a homeless shelter, or a hospital. There are always people in need of a gentle smile or a word of encouragement. The key is to reach out and share the good news of Jesus in simple acts of kindness. By our examples, we are "salt and light" to the world. (See Matthew 5:13-16)

ANONYMITY
(treating everyone with confidentiality and respect)

> Do to others what you would like them to do for
> you... (Matthew 7:12, *New Living
> Translation*)

Refraining from criticism and gossip, we accept that we
are people striving toward recovery. We are all equal in
God's eyes.

> Don't just pretend that you love others; really
> love them. Hate what is wrong. Stand on the
> side of good. Love each other with brotherly
> affection and take delight in honoring each
> other... Work happily together. Don't try to act
> big. Don't try to get into the good graces of
> important people, but enjoy the company of
> ordinary folks. And don't think you know it
> all! (Romans 12:9-10,16, *The Living Bible*)

Chapter Eleven

The Elevator is Broken—Try the Steps

God introduced me to a 12-step recovery program for my food addiction; He blessed me with freedom from compulsive overeating and food obsession. In my clarity of mind, without excess food, I began to see other areas of my life that needed healing. I welcomed the opportunity to understand God's instructions from reading his Word. *The Twelve Steps for Christians* supplied the map of the Bible for sustaining the highest quality of life, which is peaceful, happy, joyful existence on earth.

> And so, dear brothers and sisters, I plead with you to give your bodies to God. Let them be a living and holy sacrifice—the kind he will accept. When you think of what he has done for you, is this too much to ask? Don't copy the behavior and customs of this world, but let God transform you into a new person by changing the way you think. Then you will know what God wants you to do, and you will know how good and pleasing and perfect his will really is. (Romans 12:1-2, *New Living Translation*)

Acknowledgment of my powerlessness and the very real fact that I only knew what I thought I knew were my first steps to healing. As I remained free from overeating each new day, I began to see God's will in my life.

I learned how to give love and accept love.

I learned that calm, respectful tones of communication worked.

I learned the skills necessary to respond in appropriate ways when annoyances and resentments flooded my thinking.

I learned to face my fears and work through them.

I learned to replace negativity with positive, life-giving affirmations.

I learned to stop manipulating and controlling people.

I learned that people are worthy of their opinions. It was okay if someone had a different opinion than mine. It didn't make them "good" or "right" and me "bad" or "wrong."

I learned to properly and respectfully take care of myself.

I learned that inappropriate behavior was not acceptable from anyone.

I learned to accept and use criticism in a positive, constructive way.

I learned that I was worthy of love and respect.

What people thought of me was none of my business. I had to be willing to listen and admit, time and time again, that I didn't know what I didn't know.

In God's time, with His constant help, I grew to

understand and love myself as well as enjoy God's perfect plan for my life. I began to accept life on life's terms. I learned to trust God in everything, knowing that He was guiding my recovery.

The 12-step program works if you "work" it, although it is not always easy. Physical, emotional and spiritual healing requires patience, perseverance, love, understanding, commitment and accountability. You will find joy unspeakable if you apply these principles to your life. I didn't say, "You *might* find joy unspeakable." I said, "You *will* find joy unspeakable" through God's amazing grace!

If you open your hearts and minds to God's perfect plan, and focus your attention on Him, your life will continue to have more and more quality. Peace, joy and unfailing love will follow you everywhere.

> Blessed (happy, enviably fortunate, and spiritually prosperous—possessing the happiness produced by the experience of God's favor and especially conditioned by the revelation of His grace, regardless of their outward conditions) are the pure in heart, for they shall see God! [Ps.24:3,4] (Matthew 5:8, *Amplified Bible*)

The Twelve Steps and Relevant Scripture

Step 1: We admitted we were powerless over our food addiction—that our lives had become unmanageable.

> I am completely discouraged—I lie in the dust... (Psalm 119:25, *The Living Bible*)

Step 2: Came to believe that a Power greater than ourselves could restore us to sanity.

> Open my eyes to see wonderful things in your

Word. I am but a pilgrim here on earth: how I
need a map—and your commands are my chart
and guide. I long for your instructions more
than I can tell. (Psalm 119:18-20, *The Living
Bible*)

Step 3: Made a decision to turn our will and our lives over to the care of God *as we understood Him.*

Trust in the Lord with all your heart and lean not on
your own understanding; in all your ways
acknowledge him, and he will make your paths
straight. (Proverbs 3:5-6, *New International Version*)

Step 4: Made a searching and fearless moral inventory of ourselves.

Let every person carefully scrutinize *and*
examine *and* test his own conduct *and* his own
work... (Galatians 6:4, *Amplified Bible*)

Step 5: Admitted to God, to ourselves, and to another human being the exact nature of our wrongs.

Confess to one another therefore your faults
(your slips, your false steps, your offenses, your
sins) and pray [also] for one another, that you
may be healed... (James 5:16, *Amplified Bible*)

Step 6: Were entirely ready to have God remove all these defects of character.

Do not resent it when God chastens and
corrects you, for his punishment is proof of his
love. Just as a father punishes a son he
delights in to make him better, so the Lord
corrects you. (Proverbs 3:11-12, *The Living
Bible*)

Step 7: Humbly asked Him to remove our shortcomings.

> But if we confess our sins to him, he can be depended on to forgive us and to cleanse us from every wrong... (1 John 1:9, *The Living Bible*)

Step 8: Made a list of all persons we had harmed, and became willing to make amends to them all.

> Do to others as you would have them do to you. (Luke 6:31, *New International Version*)

Step 9: Made direct amends to such people wherever possible, except when to do so would injure them or others.

> Bear with each other and forgive whatever grievances you may have against one another. Forgive as the Lord forgave you. (Colossians 3:13, *New International Version*)

Step 10: Continued to take personal inventory and when we were wrong promptly admitted it.

> Now your attitudes and thoughts must all be constantly changing for the better. Yes, you must be a new and different person, holy and good. Clothe yourself with this new nature. Stop lying to each other; tell the truth, for we are parts of each other and when we lie to each other we are hurting ourselves. (Ephesians 4:23-25, *The Living Bible*)

Step 11: Sought through prayer and meditation to improve our conscious contact with God, *as we*

***understood Him*, praying only for knowledge of His will for us and the power to carry that out.**

> Pray all the time. Ask God for anything in line with the Holy Spirit's wishes. Plead with him, reminding him of your needs, and keep praying earnestly for all Christians everywhere. (Ephesians 6:18, *New Living Translation*)

Step 12: Having had a spiritual awakening as the result of these steps, we tried to carry this message to food addicts, and to practice these principles in all our affairs.

> It is God himself, in his mercy, who has given us this wonderful work [of telling his Good News to others] and so we never give up. (2 Corinthians 4:1, *The Living Bible*)

Permission to use the Twelve Steps of Alcoholics Anonymous® for adaptation granted by AA World Services, Inc.

Chapter Twelve

A Sweet Surrender

2019

The Lord is my shepherd, I shall not want. He makes me lie down in green pastures; He leads me beside quiet waters. He stores my soul: He guides me in the path of righteousness For His name's sake." (Psalm 23:1-3, *New American Standard Bible*)

Full of Faith (or full of food?)

Sometime around my 20th year anniversary of freedom from overeating, the hidden promises came true for me. My way of eating became as easy as breathing. It's who I am. It became my way of life.

> We feel as though we had been placed in a position of neutrality—safe and protected. We have not even sworn off. Instead, the problem has been removed. It does not exist for us. We are neither cocky nor are we afraid. This is our experience. That is how we react as long as we keep in fit spiritual condition. (*Alcoholics Anonymous*, page 85)

On July 23rd, 2019, I celebrated 31 years of freedom from compulsive and addictive eating, maintaining my goal weight (126-129lbs) on an ongoing basis. I am 65 years old, retired, living with my husband, Carl, in MA. Through the years, I have continued to grow in love and understanding of God's will as it applies to all aspects of my life.

God is a dream-maker. The gist of Ephesians 3:20 - "more than I could ever dare to dream, wish or imagine" - is my reality today. To God be the glory. I do not "work" to get these rewards. I sit at the feet of Jesus and am obedient by applying the disciplines of the Christian life and walking daily through the 12 steps.

My relationship with my husband continues to be my biggest challenge. Carl gives me many opportunities to practice the skills that I have learned. I try to smile in reflecting upon James' teaching. "Consider it all joy when facing trials..." (James 1:1-4), because it allows me to grow stronger in faith. Joy is not happiness, but rather an ongoing faith and trust in Jesus.

My children, their wives and my grandchildren are my most precious gifts. They love and accept me with all my shortcomings, loving as God loves them. Dan is a pastor, and Joe works as an accountant for a huge missionary organization, and they both live in Pennsylvania, only minutes away from each other, but hours from us. Dan once said, "Mom, isn't it great that we have no unfinished business?" And Joe responded to yet another amends by saying, "Mom, I hold no resentments." How sweet is that? "God, who began a good work in me, will be faithful" (Phil 1:6). My heart is filled to the brim with thanksgiving for all that the Lord has done in their lives and in the lives of their families.

"Fit spiritual condition" is the key that keeps my program "green"—alive and well. God is the answer, what's the question? I have learned to ask the Lord for help in all circumstances of my life, living day by day in close dependence on Him. Instead of telling God how big my problems are, I tell my problems how big my God is.

I am happy that I have learned to feel my feelings and now experience a full array of emotions. I cry, I laugh, and my smile is real. When I joined my first 12-step program, I not only used food to fix a feeling; I used people to fill the emptiness in my heart. My co-dependency, along with my pride and judgement, and my fear of rejection and abandonment, ruled me.

> Consider it pure joy, my brothers, whenever you face
> trials of many kinds, because you know that the
> testing of your faith develops perseverance." (James
> 1:2-3, *New International Version*)

Chapter Thirteen

Help for the Newcomer

> And let us consider how to stir up one another to love
> and good works, not neglecting to meet together, as
> is the habit of some, but encouraging one another,
> and all the more as you see the Day drawing near.
> (Hebrews 10:24-25, *New International Version*)

For the person wanting to get abstinent without yet finding a
sponsor or an accountability group, I hope to share some
insights that might help and encourage you.

In *Full of Faith*, God and abstinence are the most
important things without exception. We plan what we eat
and we eat what we plan. For the beginner in food addiction
recovery, there is our "Step Easy" suggested food plan. It is
three meals and a metabolic adjustment (a smaller
meal). There are some options for portion sizes. If you want
to lose weight, decide on the lower amounts. Please note
that we do not eat flour (this includes grain flours, nut flours,
and bean flours), sugar and other sweeteners (natural or
artificial), alcohol, snack foods (roasted nuts, popcorn or
processed grains) and dried fruit, and we weigh and measure
all our food on a food scale or using measuring cups and
spoons. We don't eat extra anything (even abstinent food),
no bites, licks or tastes.

For accountability, while trying to find a sponsor, we have a small group/thread in the Facebook *Full of Faith* Accountability group called "In Need of a Sponsor Group" (look for a graphic of a smiling face on a plate). People post their food there and one of our leaders is assigned to monitor the group each day to offer help and guidance as a temporary sponsor.

Outside everyday eating, we plan in advance for exceptional circumstances. When dining at a restaurant or at a social event, it is best to scope the scene beforehand by checking the menu online or calling to ask specific questions to be sure that our needs will be met. When we go to restaurants, we make a plan that will keep us close to our basic commitment, being 100% honest. We look for plain, pan-fried, grilled or roasted meat or fish with plain vegetables, baked potatoes and/or salad. We stay away from French fries, sauces, gravies.

For me, I order broiled steak or fish without the crumbs, baked potato, steamed vegetables and salad. I eyeball the steak or fish to the size of a deck of cards, and I cut a big baked potato in half (aiming for the visual of 1/2 cup/4 oz portion). For my fat, I use a dollop of butter (to equal one tablespoon), and I use vinegar on my salad (no oil or salad dressing), although I could choose to use oil instead of butter. Those choices are personal (Note: A tablespoon is 3 teaspoons.).

The bottom line for everyone is to not eat any sugar, flour or sweeteners and to keep the portion sizes close to normal. As a reminder, please beware that most salad dressings and condiments contain some form of sugar. For social events, it is best to call ahead to see what will be available so that you can plan how you will cope before you enter the room. It is usually wise to take back-up food with you even if it appears that there are good options. Sometimes amounts are skimpy. We don't want to feel deprived. It's a set up for failure.

There will be times when circumstances arise and you will need to change what you have planned. For emergency dining (those times when you thought you'd be home, but aren't), you could eat at a fast-food chain being careful to order with a plan in mind. For me, I order a burger (without the bun), a salad (dry) and a baked potato (if I am at a Wendy's), using butter as the fat for the meal. Since my salad is minimal, I would eat 3/4 of the potato instead. Again, if you are opting for a salad dressing instead of butter, always check the labels. If I cannot get a potato, then I buy a fruit for the meal. Fries or potato puffs are not an option for us. It is important to always tell someone what you are doing and why. It's the motive that matters.

Getting sick, and therefore unable to eat normally, causes us to change our intended plan for the day. I usually have a couple of options for these kinds of days. One option is to have breakfast again for lunch or dinner; another option is to have a simple homemade vegetable and chicken/fish soup that is easy to prepare and gentle on the stomach. Having a plan for these exceptions is what matters most. We don't want to rationalize and justify our "need" to eat off plan. Having these back-up plans in place assures that we will be abstinent no matter what happens. Again, when this happens, we tell another food addict, so that we are not alone in any decision.

There are times when we go to get something that we had planned to eat only to find out that it has spoiled or has disappeared because a family member ate it. These situations can also be challenging. When they inevitably occur, we make equal exchanges, but with the 100% honesty approach - we tell someone. You can write on the accountability group, text or call a fellow member. We don't keep any secrets about our food.

When I set out on a new day, I think of all the possibilities, and I either bring food with me or know what I will do in different situations. I often carry my metabolic adjustment (could be referred to as a "snack") for those times when I need to rearrange the order of my meals.

These suggestions may sound complicated, but it is important to remember that planning is essential. I have heard and confirmed through personal experience that "the person who fails to plan, plans to fail."

A Life-Giving Program

Whenever temptations plague us, as they undoubtedly will, there are things we do to help us make it through the thoughts, wants, and feelings for more food. We often compare these action steps to instruments in a tool box. They equip us in building a strong foundation. The cornerstone is Jesus. Extra food is NOT in our tool boxes.

Communication with God and other members is first and foremost. We communicate with our fellow members by phone calls, texts, emails or personal messages. We share how we feel and/or ask how fellow food addicts survive from meal to meal.

Attending phone meetings keeps us connected. Members share their experience, strength and hope, and even their struggles.

Reading the *Life Recovery Bible*, The Big Book (*Alcoholics Anonymous*) and *The Twelve Steps for Christians* can all help us to understand the intricacies of recovery and identify the things in our lives that draw us out of God's will and purpose. It is the truth that sets us free - the process of realization, acceptance and surrender.

Writing posts on the Facebook group pages, journaling our feelings, and participating in step studies are good ways to replace our food thoughts. Food never fixes a problem or a feeling. Peer pressure can seem unbearable at times, but we need to dispel the myth that we are normal when it comes to food. We are "normal" in these rooms. In fact, we are our best selves when we are in recovery.

All the tools we practice are part of an intentional action plan. Committing a food plan each day, participating in the online groups and/or at a meeting, making phone calls, praying for others in the group are all actions we take as part of making the choice to stay abstinent, which is defined as following our food plans no matter what is happening in our circumstances or how we feel.

Finally, working the 12 steps is vital. Abstinence is the zero step. Steps 1-12 are the life-changing process of transformation/restoration. In my head and heart, the first three steps are "I cannot control my eating; my life is a mess (Step One), God and people who have gone before me can help me (Step Two). I will let them (Step Three)." Here's the prayer that I memorized on my first day of abstinence:

> God, I offer myself to Thee-
> To build with me
> and to do with me as Thou wilt.
> Relieve me of the bondage of self,
> that I may better do Thy will.
> Take away my difficulties,
> that victory over them may bear witness
> to those I would help of Thy Power,
> Thy Love, and Thy Way of life.
> May I do Thy will always!

The Third Step Prayer from page 63 of the Big Book, *Alcoholics Anonymous*.
Copyright © Alcoholics Anonymous World Services, Inc.

My mantra has carried me through many storms...use as needed...

> My food is my food. *Everything else is not my food.* It is not an option to overeat *no matter what* is happening in my circumstances or how I feel.

Period. End of food thought. Love and service keeps me dry.

Love and service is doing whatever I need to do to stay free and clean. We apply all these principles "Just for today." We don't worry about tomorrow, our birthday or the next holiday or vacation.

So don't be anxious about tomorrow. God will take care of your tomorrow, too. Live one day at a time. (Matt 6:33, *The Living Bible*)

This is our *Full of Faith* greeting.
(Different people respond by saying the next line.)

It is a brand new day to rejoice and be glad!
God's mercies are new every morning!
The Lord is my shepherd; I have everything that I need.
The joy of the Lord is my strength.
Toe bump; *you* matter!

Chapter Fourteen

Farewell—Follow the Cloud

> Jesus told them, "I assure you, even if you had faith as
> small as a mustard seed, you could say to this
> mountain, 'Move from here to there,' and it would
> move. Nothing would be impossible." (Matthew
> 17:20, *New Living Translation*)

This is *a rich and rewarding new way of life*. When you make
the decision to follow a committed plan of eating, it is possible
to stay abstinent and free from compulsive overeating and
food obsession. Your new mindset will replace the old self-
destructive tapes that once controlled your life. Start with
words like "I think I can. I think I can. I think I can."

God wants us to be happy, and He wants us to
succeed. The momentum will flow. Do your 1%, which is
following a food plan, and God will carry you from
there. Soon you will be saying, "Thank you, Jesus, for
another day of abstinence." If you can find the willingness to
join me in recovery, you will find a peace and clarity that
passes all understanding.

God bless you as you consider this difficult, yet life-
changing challenge. Visit our website: www.fulloffaith.com

and join our private Facebook groups for personal interaction, support and encouragement. You would be welcomed.

> God is faithful. "...God, who began the good work within you, will continue his work until it is finally finished..." (Philippians 1:6, *New Living Translation*)

Testimonies

HOPE—Hearing Other People's Experiences

As a testimony of God's love and grace, some *Full of Faith* members wanted to share their experience, strength and hope with you.

Hilary from the UK

(co-facilitator)

Hello, my name is Hilary and I live in the UK. This is my story.

22nd May 2014 was the date God set my feet on a new pathway that has changed my life. To explain I need to backtrack to my childhood. I knew at quite an early age that I had an issue with food. Normal children knew when they were hungry and when to stop eating; my body did not work like that and at times I ate far more than I needed, helping myself to things from cupboards at home and even taking money from my mother's purse so I could go to the shop on the way home from school. I knew this was not right and I did not like it, but could not stop it.

When, as a teenager, I became a Christian I knew this did not please God either. What I read in the Bible told me this was not the way He wanted His child to behave. I swallowed my pride on three occasions as a young Christian and asked for help from people I trusted, but each one thought I was worried about my weight when in fact this was a far greater burden than extra pounds. So, I shut it away in my life where I thought no one could see it and coped with it as best I could on my own. I was so ashamed!

I prayed about it often, asked God, cried out to Him, even begged Him to take the strong cravings away, but still they continued. I asked for will power to withstand the cravings and at times I could control them, but at other times they controlled me. I tried all sorts of things to try and get free, but nothing worked. I often felt it was like being an alcoholic, but with food as the problem substance. How I envied alcoholics the fact that they could put the stopper on the bottle. There did not seem to be a way for me to do that as I had no option but to eat every day.

In early 2014 I came to a point of despair, having come to the conclusion that I was not going to find an answer this side of the grave. I knew my life was crippled by this emotionally, mentally, and spiritually as well as physically. I was depressed and could not get any relief. In desperation I went searching the internet and found, to my surprise, that there was indeed such a condition as food addiction; that scientists had shown that for some people certain foods were toxic causing chemical reactions in the brain producing powerful cravings in just the same way as alcohol can do.

Adding "Christian" to "Food addiction" on Google brought me to *Full of Faith* and my life changed. I read every word on the website and knew straight away that God had brought me to the answer I had been seeking for over 50 years. I learned that the substances that caused my cravings were the refined carbohydrates and for someone with this condition one bite of any food containing sugar or flour had the potential to cause major problems.

With hope in my heart I prayed about this and God gave me a picture. It was of a dungeon, there was a figure inside cowering in a corner, but the door was open and light was flooding in where for so many years there had been gloom and darkness. He showed me that I was that figure. To be free all I had to do was get up and walk out.

That sounded simple. However, I knew eating without flour and sugar for the rest of my life was an enormous step, but this was a life and death moment for me. So, 22nd May 2014 was the day I handed it all over to God. I planned my meals carefully with no flour or sugar and I ate what I had planned and nothing else. I got up and tentatively walked out of the dungeon of food addiction ...to a life of freedom.

Today I am still on the pathway. One day at a time, by the grace of God and with His strength, I stick to my daily food plan. One day at a time is all God asks. I haven't got to worry about tomorrow until it comes. The dungeon is still there with its open door and I know that with just one bite I would be back on the inside. I don't want to go there. Freedom is wonderful. My life has been changing in every way since May 2014. Physically, emotionally, mentally and spiritually God has been healing this crippled life as I have worked through the 12-steps with Pam's leading.

I am no longer hiding - now I can be real.

I am no longer dependent on food to satisfy my emotional needs - now I am free.

I am no longer in despair - now I have hope.

I am no longer struggling to cope - now I am learning to live.

And I could add many, many more benefits of walking this pathway.

I am so grateful to God for bringing me to where I am today - to Him be the glory! God has been growing a desire in my heart to help others and to share the good news that there is a way to live that brings freedom from food addiction. I particularly have a heart for people in the UK who are suffering, as I was for so long, and have not found the information they need to set their feet on the pathway to freedom.

I am happy and excited to be supporting Pam and the other ministry leaders in bringing this life-changing ministry to the food addicts of the world.   Hilary from the UK

Ann from MA

Hi! My name is Ann from MA. I am a compulsive overeater. I have been on the diet go-round for as long as I can remember. When I was about six years old, I remember sitting on cellar stairs with a group of kids eating cookies. For some reason, I hid my cookies, telling them I was done. I may have thought they would give me theirs if they saw that I didn't have any. I do not know.

During my teenage years, I shopped with my Mom and bought all kinds of snacks. When we got home, she relaxed with a beer, and I relaxed with junk food. I needed to eat whatever snacks we bought. I started with one bowl of one snack, then opened the next bag or box and served myself another bowl. Almost as if I was taste testing, I continued to open each new package or container until I had sampled the full array of our new supply.

When I was about 13, I went on my first diet, "The Grapefruit Diet." It wasn't a diet that suited my life-style, so I continued my search. After seeing our family's physician, I tried Weight Watchers, Jenny Craig, Dexitrim, and other diet pills on the market. I counted calories, tried Atkins, Special K Diet, Slim Fast, Medifast, South Beach, and I often read a new magazine and tried "The diet of the week." I tried a diet where I ate certain foods on certain days and fasted on other days. I tried dieting all week and then having treats on the weekend. For me, that just reversed my week of hard work. I went to a couple of nutritionists. Some of these diets worked for a short time, but not for long.

I came to believe that my husband was right when he said, "DIET is DIE with a T." I once thought that I'd be able to eat like a "normal" person once I lost my excess weight, but after

181

40 years of dieting, and 40 years of discouragement, having made the scale my report card, I needed a LIFETIME CHANGE. I needed to create new habits and new mindsets. I didn't need to find a way that would bring me back to my old way of eating.

Why did I want to lose weight? To look good? To feel good? To get in those jeans that I love? Upcoming wedding or event? Those are temporary reasons, but the best and long lasting reason is to attain and maintain a healthy body, physically, emotionally, spiritually.

I CANNOT DO WHAT I DID BEFORE, AND EXPECT DIFFERENT RESULTS.

From 2009 to August 2018, I lost and gained over 200 lbs., 9 years of my journey. In April 2017, I joined *Full of Faith* weighing 164 lbs. My current weight is 123 lbs. I am the healthiest I have ever been. July 2019 I will be 62, and I am medication free.

To be honest, I came to *Full of Faith* to lose weight. I now realize that being overweight was a tool God used to get my attention. The tool box in *Full of Faith*, the daily disciplines, have taught me how to live in faithful surrender.

I pray that you will be encouraged to join us in recovery. Thank you. Ann from MA

Julie from OR

Hi, my name is Julie from Oregon, a Christian in recovery from food addiction.

At a young age, I remember finding comfort in food. When I was sad, frightened, bored, you name it, I turned to food. I was diagnosed with diabetes at age 18. I did not want to be different from my friends, so I went to my go-to for handling stress or painful experiences. My go-to was more food. Avoidance and denial, along with the food, were my coping skills. Therefore, I avoided and denied my diagnosis of diabetes for 10 years.

At age 30, because of blurred vision, I was sent to a retina specialist. I had two intrusive surgeries on my eyes to remove scar tissue, caused by uncontrolled diabetes, along with numerous laser surgeries. The surgeries did not work, therefore, I lost complete vision in both eyes. At this time, my weight increased to 250 pounds.

Around a year prior to joining *Full of Faith*, I was convicted by God that my eating was not pleasing to Him and the battle began with the cycle of promises to God to "do better" tomorrow, and the guilt, shame and hopelessness that followed when I could not fulfill that promise. I would do okay for breakfast and lunch on most days, but when dinner came, I just did not/could not stop overeating.

I had a friend on Facebook who posted that she had been clean from drugs for three years and I thought to myself, "I cannot stop bingeing for one day." I had never even heard of food addiction before, but decided to google it and found *Full of Faith*. I read the distinctives for *Full of Faith* and thought "I can't do this." I prayed to God to help me, my first step of surrender. I had an ounce of willingness. God took that seed of willingness and caused it to grow.

My journey in *Full of Faith* has not been perfect; it took me many months to get consecutive days of following my committed food plan, but by God's grace, I have 2 1/2 years of back-to-back abstinence. I want to share some of the changes I have experienced since beginning in *Full of Faith* almost three years ago. Physically, emotionally and spiritually, my life has changed as a byproduct of abstinence and surrender.

Physical Changes

When I started the program, I was taking 90 units of a

slow acting insulin twice a day and up to 200 units of fast acting insulin a day, as well as six different prescription medications for diabetes, blood pressure, high cholesterol and depression. My hemoglobin A1C was way above normal, and I had a lot of trouble sleeping, only getting about 4 hours of sleep per night, which led to exhaustion, fatigue and relationship problems.

Fast forward three years, there is no longer a need for me to take insulin. I only take two prescription medications. My blood pressure, hemoglobin A1C, and cholesterol are all within normal ranges. I actually get to sleep a full 7-8 hours a night, and after losing between 120 and 125 pounds, my weight is, for the first time in my life, within a healthy range and BMI.

None of these things would have been possible without God. It isn't my will power that has gotten me through these changes, but my daily surrender to His will; God has done in me what I have never been able to do for myself. "In my weakness He is strong."

Emotional Changes

Emotionally, I was struggling with guilt, isolation, shame, self-loathing and depression. Most often I felt frozen and in a mental fog. I buried my emotions with food, not allowing myself to feel and deal with them, which left me irritable and, at times, irrational.

Now, I can find joy in Christ because I am not drowning in my undealt with emotions. I've been given the daily disciplines and the 12 steps and willingness to work through my emotions in a God-honoring way, instead of avoiding and denying them. It isn't always easy, but God has been revealing to me how unhealthy I was. He is showing me the lies that I believed about myself, Him, and others. He is taking me through many fears that have plagued me for most of my life and is giving me the ability to finally find healing and joy. It has been, and still is, a process of the Word of God becoming instilled in my heart, not just knowledge in my head, as I surrender to Him.

"He who loses his life will gain it." It is progress not perfection. "As a child I acted as a child." Before beginning this process, I didn't realize how dead I was emotionally by trying to cling to my fears. But God is showing me a more abundant life and healing as I surrender my emotions to Him.

Spiritual Changes

I felt lost in a perpetual desert, distant from God, desiring to be close and honest with Him, but finding myself always falling short. I didn't know what I didn't know. I was in the Word daily, thinking I was growing, but I was deceiving myself by not allowing the Word to do its work in me. I was "being a hearer only." I abused the grace God gave me by knowing what I was doing was wrong, but doing it anyway. Because I knew I could find forgiveness, I was unwilling to lay down my idol of food.

Daily surrendering to God through working the 12 steps as a way of life, I am finding submission in other areas of my life becoming easier and habitual. By practicing discipline by weighing and measuring my food, I have become more disciplined in my spiritual walk. Being willing to let go of the food idol has released me from the burdens and walls that I had put up between myself and God.

I feel awakened to the Holy Spirit and His leading. "Draw near to God and he will draw near to you." I've moved my walk with Christ from a checklist of "do" and "don't" to an intimacy with God and a real desire to just be in the presence of God. Surrendering to God has been my path to healing. Julie from OR

Kevin from CA

I can remember food being my friend as far back as grade school. I could never get enough and it didn't seem to matter what I was eating. My mom and dad struggled financially to support four kids, so we took bag lunches to school. My mom would buy boxes of treats to put in our lunch boxes, and we had an extra freezer in the garage where she stored these goodies. I raided that freezer often, eating frozen sweet treats by the boxful. She knew it was happening, but with four kids she didn't know who was to blame for the missing stash. If she would have thought about it, she would have known it was the chubby 3rd grader with the evidence smeared around his lips. Hey, I was in the 3rd grade! My hiding skills weren't perfected yet.

When I was around 10 years old, school was a miserable experience for me. I was shy, awkward and uncoordinated, the kind of kid I have major compassion for today. One evening I came home feeling really upset about my weight. In my family of origin, communication flowed like dry cement, so I bit the bullet and approached it the easy way by writing my mom a note telling her how much I wanted to lose weight. I told her that I was tired of being teased.

I left the note on the kitchen table and waited. And waited. And waited. I knew she had found it, but she never talked to me about it. In my 10-year old mind, I equated that with shame. My mom was too ashamed to even broach the subject with me. At that point I had perfected my hiding skills. I was stealing things from the refrigerator, stealing money to buy snacks, eating my Halloween stash and then eating my siblings' treats. I was good at sneaking food. Unfortunately, that skill followed me into high school, college and beyond.

In my senior year of high school, I found myself living alone in a motel room because I refused to move with my family for the umpteenth time. My parents and siblings moved, but I stayed. I had a job at a local fast food restaurant and kept up my dysfunctional eating there, stuffing my pockets with food to take back to the motel. I can remember getting paid and spending the whole paycheck on junk food at the convenience store attached to the motel. Eating until I was sick, depressed, lonely and even suicidal.

At this point in time, I met Jesus and my life took a turn in the right direction. The suicidal thoughts stopped, but my overeating didn't. Therefore, I added guilt to my backpack of shortcomings. I loved God and I was growing spiritually, but I couldn't stop overeating. As a result, my health suffered significantly. I was diagnosed with diabetes and it took its toll on me. Amputations of toes and finally a foot, kidney failure, eye problems leading to blindness in one eye, two heart attacks and uncontrolled blood sugar followed. All of this was still not enough for me to give up my overeating or my right to eat junk food.

I was introduced to *Full of Faith* through my sister's experience. I watched her journey of weight loss and witnessed her strides in getting healthier, so I asked what she was doing. She introduced me to *Full of Faith*. It wasn't an easy answer for me. The first time I heard the term "food addict," I actually laughed, "How can you be addicted to food?" I found a quiz for food addiction online and answered the questions. Sure enough, there in black and white was the answer. I am a food addict. I answered 10 out of 10 questions with a "yes." Go figure. I messaged Pam and started on my journey to recovery.

I found strength, hope and encouragement in the *Full of Faith* community and lost my excess weight. People warned me that maintenance is where the rubber hits the road, but I didn't understand what that meant until it was too late. I got cocky and pride snuck its way into my thinking. After two months of abstinence, I figured "I've got this," and decided to ease up on my food plan. I "woke up" about a year later back where I started. I humbled myself and asked to be added back to the Facebook groups again, because I had deleted all of the group pages. I was graciously welcomed back and have been on a steady upswing ever since. The difference came when I got serious about Step Three. God can, and I'll let Him.

My program is strong today because I know now what I didn't know then. It's about daily surrender. My blood sugars are in tight control and I have drastically decreased the amount of medicine I take.

My hope for the future is that I will continue this journey, sharing the incredible freedom found as a result of abstinence. I am thankful that God is opening doors of opportunities that excite me. There's a world of hurting people out there and for His honor, I pray that I might have the privilege of walking alongside them as they discover the freedom that I have found in *Full of Faith*. I am a grateful believer in Jesus in recovery from food addiction. Kevin from CA

Angie from GA

I began sneaking food and overeating at the age of five. I wasn't a heavy child or teenager because I was involved in physical activities, but I would secretly sneak food at my grandparent's house, babysitting jobs, other workplaces and in my locked bedroom. Throughout my life I learned that I needed to sneak food to avoid embarrassment. I was confused as to how I could be a Christian who prays, asks for God's help and forgiveness, yet overeat again and again. I lacked the self-control, discipline and commitment that the Bible talks about. One night after yet another binge, I went online and typed "Christian food addiction" in the search box. I clicked on *Full of Faith* and learned about the science of food addiction, that I wasn't alone, that there is a solution. Although I immediately eliminated trigger foods, I wasn't dealing with my emotions on a daily basis, so I continued to overeat. Until I walked through the 12 steps, I still believed the lie, without realizing it, that food would fix my problems. Because I gained and lost the same few pounds over and over again, it gave me the illusion of control and kept me in denial. I was still considering food as an option to be used for comfort and as an escape from reality.

I had what felt like a million "day ones." I could stop overeating, but I couldn't stay stopped. I was scared to leave program because I knew my life would be in ruins, yet my relapse cycle was insane. I tried a lot of external things to fix me, new food plans, new sponsors, other recovery groups, new step studies, new books and more, but I could not achieve long-term abstinence. I was also a slave to the bathroom scale and used it to gauge my worth and value. I realize now that this was another form of denial. If I stayed under a certain weight, I rationalized that what I was doing was okay.

After sharing my struggles with members of *Full of Faith*, I was lovingly confronted by a friend in the ministry who suggested I write about what I really wanted from recovery. I learned that I wanted the benefits of program, but I also wanted the food as my escape hatch. I wrestled with God about this, as I knew I had to make a big-picture, life-long decision. Was I all in or all out? I couldn't keep straggling the barbed-wire fence of addiction. I was angry to have these food issues and scared to give up the food and be "done". After three days and reaching the point of exhaustion, I said, "Okay, God, I know You are faithful and I'm having trouble trusting You with this, but I'm going to have a mustard seed of faith and be done with the food." I was immediately washed with peace and relief.

During the first three days, God repeatedly gave me a scripture (Galatians 2:20) that described how it felt to crucify my old self through surrender and be risen anew with Jesus. I took that as my mantra. Each time I experienced a food thought, a rationalization, or any negative self-talk, I would think or say, "No! I'm done! Food is not an option. It is no longer I who live, but Christ who lives within me. The life I live now is a life of faith. I completely trust You, Jesus." Amazingly, this practice renewed my mind and rewired my thinking time after time.

Deciding to be "done" with the food was a big-picture decision, but I have to live it out moment by moment, one day at a time. The things that help me maintain long-term abstinence are:

- The decision to be done with the food, which has simplified my thinking and encourages me to utilize the tools of *Full of Faith* for support, gets me out of myself, and creates depth in my relationship with God.

- Intentional time with the Lord and total dependence on Him moment by moment. I ask Him for help, then I thank Him each time He helps me. This practice takes my self-reliance and pride out of the picture. I, also, process any distorted concepts I have of God that hinder me from connecting with Him. His character is not the same as a human's, so I need to continually recognize that fact and separate the two.

- Having a list of the lies and thoughts that precede the first bite for me. Then, when those thoughts pop up in real time, I recognize they are lies, reject and replace them with truth.

- Practicing self-awareness, and I am learning to process normal emotions, so that they don't build up and drive me to the food. Since I wasn't familiar with recognizing when I was uncomfortable, I set my phone to remind me several times a day to ask, "Is something bothering me?" I process any negative responses as soon as possible using the 12 steps found in the Big Book and through prayer. Then I replace self-centered thoughts with ways that I can be helpful to others.

- Working the tools of *Full of Faith* on a daily basis has become automatic. Rather than considering it a checklist, each tool creates depth in my relationship with God and with others. Several of the tools involve service to others, which is a big part of keeping my recovery strong.

Putting the food down gave me neutrality from physical cravings, but the Big Book of AA says the bigger problem is in the mind. The tools, steps and thinking patterns all guided by God and His power, help me heal from the inside out. One day at a time I pray to keep growing and enjoying this wonderful life of recovery. I am so thankful!! Angie in GA

Cathy from NH

"The Lord is my shepherd; I shall not want." I read that and even memorized the 23rd Psalm in my younger years. I was a Christian yet struggled and felt defeated most of the time, because of my ongoing war with food. For over 40 years, I was either dieting or overeating. I tried diet pills, fad programs, bought the books, shakers and matching utensils, the mixes, ordered the boxes, met with a nutritionist, joined clubs and went to meetings, all to no avail. I couldn't stay on any diet for long. My yo-yo dieting/overeating continued until I resolved to just be overweight for the rest of my life.

People consoled me with, "you have a pretty face," so I hid behind those words and stayed in denial about the severity of my condition. My eyes opened when I bought some cute summer tops to wear on a trip to Florida and saw the pictures taken on that trip. I hardly recognized myself in those pictures! Knowing my doctor had cautioned me about my hypertension, high cholesterol and overweight stats just confirmed that it was time for a change.

Easter Sunday arrived shortly thereafter. In my Sunday kids' class, 6 yr old Liam came bounding in all excited and exclaimed "JESUS HAS THE POWER." The morning was full of celebration of God's goodness and Jesus' Resurrection! On my way home from church that morning, my eyes filled with tears. I cried out, "Lord, where is Your power in my life?" Looking back, I'm still not quite sure of the chain of events, but I remember seeing an ad for a 12-step weight loss solution. I looked into it and was introduced to the science of food addiction, a food plan that brings freedom from food cravings, and an awareness of eating behaviors and how to handle emotions.

I started to dabble and debate with the ideas presented, as I continued my search. I wanted a biblical approach to support me. Psalm 23:3 says "He restores my soul. He leads me in paths of righteousness for His name's sake." I wanted this time to be different. I wanted to change, really change. I found Pam's book, *Sweet Surrender,* and felt like I had found the missing link. I joined *Full of Faith* and claimed April 1, 2017, as the day that I quit fooling myself and accepted I was a compulsive overeater and food addict. *Full of Faith* was the last house on the block for me! Finally home, I began my journey in recovery.

Psalm 23:4 says, "God is with me and His rod and staff comfort me." It took me about a year to lose 65 lbs. During that time, I felt God's leading, guidance and provision in new and exciting ways. Because I stopped using food to cover-up emotions, I learned healthier ways to deal with them. With the help of my *Full of Faith* family, I discovered that surrender, acceptance, gratitude, contentment and joy are just some of the place settings at the table the Lord has prepared for me where defeat, doubt, distrust and dysfunction once sat.

I had never been at my goal weight for more than a couple of days in all my 40+ years of yo-yo dieting/overeating, however, God changed me! I have maintained a 65 lb. weight loss for over a year! My doctor is amazed. I'm off all medications for high blood pressure and high cholesterol. I live life in a whole new way. I enjoy being active, even tap dancing classes, and I like not having to store three sizes of clothes in my closet. Ps 23:6 "Surely God's goodness and mercy follow me!" God has changed my life through the *Full of Faith* ministry. Cathy from NH

Christine from MA

My name is Christine. I am 56 years old and have been a food addict since a very early age, probably birth! I remember being so small that I was looking up at the counter while stealing food. Up until the age of 12, my mother controlled what I ate and I was a normal body weight. Two things happened to change that. First, my mother got a job. I had full access to the pantry and could eat what I wanted when I wanted it. Second, my dad's friend who owned a pig farm started showing up at our house with a dump truck full of all kinds of refined snack and dessert foods that he had access to because they had just passed their "sell by" dates, therefore, we had a never-ending supply of junk food that was free. My bingeing days began.

I had a lot of anxiety as a child and I didn't know what to do with it. Food helped to relieve the anxiety. The latest science in the arena of food addiction shows that the same reward and pleasure centers in the brain that are triggered by addictive drugs like heroin and cocaine are also activated by ultra-refined and highly palatable foods rich in sugars, flours, fats, and salt. Like addictive drugs, these foods trigger feel-good chemicals like dopamine. I learned to turn to these foods when I felt any uncomfortable feelings. Unfortunately, just like with addictive drugs, the more a person uses something to attempt to relieve feelings, the less it will work and the more they will need. This is where I found myself at a young age. I ate more and it worked less, requiring me to keep increasing the amount I ate.

When I was 26, I was introduced to a 12-step program for compulsive overeating. I used the program as a diet to lose weight for my wedding. As soon as the wedding day hit, the diet was over. I left the program and started gaining back the weight. By my first anniversary, I was pregnant with my son and was eating as if I was pregnant with quadruplets! After the delivery of my son, I found myself scared because I couldn't stop eating, so I made my way back to the only diet that had ever worked for me. I followed the food plan from the 12-step program, and I lost 90 pounds in 6 months, but again left the program once my weight was down. This began decades of working the food plan in the program, but not much else, until my weight was down. Then I'd leave and come back when I was out of control and had gained back all of my weight and more. It was a vicious cycle. In 1995, I gave my life to the Lord and in subsequent years, I tried many Christian weight-loss programs with the same effect.

Fast-forward to 2016, I found myself in dire circumstances. My bingeing was so out of control; it was all I could do all day. I was struggling in my relationship with the Lord, mired in shame and disgust with myself because I would promise Him that this was the day that I was going to give it all up. Just hours later, I would feel so uncomfortable in my feelings and because of withdrawal, I would find myself running to the food. It felt like a hand came out of the pit of hell, grabbed me by the jugular, and held me down. I would read scriptures like, "I can do all things through Christ who strengthens me," and wonder what was wrong with me.

In June of 2016, I started working the *Full of Faith* program, but this time I caught the vision that this was about so much more than a diet! When I looked at the tools and steps of the program, I saw that they were leading me to live the life of devotion to the Lord that I had desired to live for a long time. The Lord showed me that turning to food in my times of stress was actually idolatry and a poor substitute for what I really needed, which was Him. I needed to pray, read His Word, meditate upon it, and seek direction for my day (Tools of Literature, Prayer and Meditation, and Action Plan). I needed to lay down those foods that triggered the release of dopamine and other feel-good chemicals and turn to Him alone. I did this by following the Step Easy food plan and committing my food to a sponsor (Tools of Abstinence and Accountability). I needed to reach out via phone, private message or text to other believers in *Full of Faith*. I needed to attend phone meetings each day to encourage others and to receive encouragement. I learned the truth of the saying, "Together we can do what we could never do alone." (Tools of Communication, Meetings, and Love and Service). I needed to inventory my life to see where I was living out of God's will.

> Search me, O God, and know my heart; test me and know my anxious thoughts. Point out anything in me that offends you, and lead me along the path of everlasting life. (Ps 139:23-24)

As a child, I had learned two coping mechanisms: stuffing down my feelings and eating food to relieve anxiety. I had to learn new godly and healthy coping mechanisms (12 Step Study and Writing). I learned that what was needed was a whole life change, not just a diet.

It is good news that God is in the business of changing lives and that is what He did for me. Over the years, I had wondered why God would not answer my prayers over my bingeing and excess weight. I realized that He wanted to bless me with so much more than weight loss. He was waiting until I was willing to, as the Third Step says, turn my will and my life over to Him. I needed to get off the throne and yield it to the One to whom it belonged! *Full of Faith* is about so much more than weight loss. It is about having a right relationship with Him with no idols! It is about becoming the people He created us to be so that we can do the good works He prepared for us long ago.

> For we are God's masterpiece. He has created us anew in Christ Jesus, so we can do the good things He planned for us long ago. (Ephesians 2:10)

So many blessings have come since the day I began to work the *Full of Faith* program on June 6th, 2016. I have the relationship with God that I have longed for since I began my walk with Him. My marriage, which suffered greatly through my years of bingeing, has been restored. I have been blessed by having my husband join me in this program. I have learned to deal with all of the challenges of life in a healthy, godly manner. I have learned to eat nutritious whole foods in the right amounts and have lost 50 lbs. My life has been transformed. In the end, God answered all of my prayers by leading me to *Full of Faith*. I have experienced the "sweet surrender" and never desire to go back. If you find yourself in the same situation I was in, take heart. There is hope. You will find help and encouragement by joining us in *Full of Faith*. Christine from MA

Doug from MA

My name is Doug, I'm a food addict. I didn't have a problem with food until I was 13. It was a challenging year because my mom had developed schizophrenia and was often emotionally unstable and my father had anger issues. They set each other off. That summer, I wasn't fitting in with the neighborhood kids, so I spent most of my time alone at home, which was a very tough place to be. My mother was a horrible cook. She was the first to admit it. It was common for her to either cook food until it nearly burst into flames or undercook it so it was still cold in the pan. Every meal was a culinary adventure! With time on my hands and out of pure survival, I taught myself to cook. I cooked a lot and ate a lot that summer. Food was one of the few things that I could control. It brought me temporary comfort and peace in a hostile environment. My compulsive eating had begun and I started to gain weight, but I played football when I entered high school, so the increased activity helped me lose most of the weight I had gained that summer.

When I turned 16, I stopped playing football and took a job at a sub shop to earn money for college. I had access to a lot of food and since my activity level had dropped significantly, my weight started climbing again. As my waistline expanded, I never saw myself as being overweight. I was just a "big guy." My size never hindered me physically, it never affected my work or my social life, and it didn't mean much besides bigger clothes. I took pride in being a "big guy." In college, my weight went up even more. Unlimited amounts of starchy food served buffet style for free, combined with sedentary studying, meant much bigger clothes than ever before. In my mind, I was still playing sports and weighing 185 lbs., but in reality, I was eating football-sized meals with snacks in between and was over 260 lbs.

Just before graduating, I met a feisty Irish woman and fell in love. We became eating buddies and both of us began steadily gaining even more weight. We loved each other and we loved eating food. Within a year, I reached my highest weight of 285 lbs. Our wedding was approaching and we wanted to lose weight, so we joined Weight Watchers. After a few months, we switched to a 12-step program for compulsive overeating because it was free. I lost over 90 lbs.! With my weight loss success, I thought I was cured and could eat whatever I wanted again. This began a cycle of losing and regaining weight, repeating this same cycle 3-4 times over the next 20 years. Every holiday, every family gathering, every anything was a reason to celebrate with food. I even celebrated weight loss with food! Providing lots of food meant I was a good provider, right? Being overweight more often than not, I convinced myself that I was just a big person. It was in my genes, my fate in life. So many lies!

I didn't have any relationship with God until my son was born. My wife and I decided we wanted to raise him with a religious background of some kind. Neither of us liked the churches we came from, so we began to search for God together over the next couple of years and we found Him! Accepting Christ was life-changing for all of us, but due to my consuming relationship with food, my relationship waxed and waned with God. As my food addiction progressed and my weight yo-yo'd up and down over the years, my relationships with my wife, children, co-workers and family suffered, too. At my worst, I was 285 lbs., full of anger, distant from God and on the verge of divorce. At my best, I was "only" mildly obese at 210 lbs., attended church but had no real relationship with God, and somewhat peacefully co-existed with my wife. I was not growing or thriving. I was not the man I wanted to be. I was not living the life I wanted to live.

Over the years, we gained and lost together, found success and failure together, sometimes helping and often hindering each other along the way. Each time I failed, my addiction grew worse. I've been blessed with an amazing godly wife who recognized her food addiction and sought recovery. In 2016, she found abstinence in *Full of Faith*. She experienced the "sweet surrender." I witnessed her change, not just with her weight loss, but in her relationships with God, me, our sons and the people around her. It was beautiful. I saw other *Full of Faith* people changing their lives, growing and thriving with years of victory over food addiction, and I wanted what they had. I *really* wanted what they had. It took six months but I finally came to see that addiction was destroying my mental, physical and spiritual health and I didn't want to live that way anymore. It was time for me to do what they did, so I could have what they had.

I came to see my addiction as sin. "...Sin is crouching at the door, eager to control you. But you must subdue it and be its master." (Genesis 4:7) Food was the "thorn in my flesh." (2 Corinthians 12:7-10) No one could do this for me. I didn't have the strength to do it for myself. It could not be a diet this time. God had to be involved in and through it all for me to truly beat my addiction.

In December of 2016, I admitted I was powerless. I put my food on God's altar and surrendered it and my will to Him. I started following the Step Easy Plan for Men and committing my food to a sponsor. In the beginning, I experienced strong food cravings and was hanging on one day at a time, but I prayed and faithfully read the Bible every day, no exceptions. I kept a book of key scriptures that strengthened me. I also kept a journal to record things that reinforced my abstinence. I listened to meetings and kept coming back. I gave up more abstinent foods because they were triggers for me. I joined an accountability group for men in *Full of Faith* and I fellowshipped with recovering addicts.

After a few months, I became food neutral for the first time in my life. Six months after surrendering to Him, I had lost 65 lbs. and gained a real relationship with my Lord and Savior Jesus Christ. I am down 100 lbs. from my top weight. I have gained stronger relationships with my wife and children. I have learned to manage my problems without using food. Today, I continue to grow and thrive as He intends for me to do. Every day I'm getting healthier mentally, physically and spiritually and helping others to do the same. To God be the glory! Doug from MA

Elizabeth from MA

My name is Elizabeth. I am a recovering food addict, solely by the grace of God. My story starts in my young teens. I tried Weight Watchers as early as 12 or 13 years of age. I was only ten or fifteen pounds overweight, but I felt unacceptable, not good enough. My mom and her entire family were very overweight, and I think Mom was trying to help me avoid the same scenario by emphasizing the importance of physical appearance. Therefore, I struggled through high school wanting to be one of the thin cheerleader types, the popular girls, and even though I was only 10 or 15 pounds overweight, I never felt acceptable. At the end of high school and during the beginning of college, I had a car, so I made a lot of stops at fast food places and did a lot of eating away from home.

I met my husband at my high school graduation. A friend had fixed us up. My father was away working and could not make it to the ceremony, but here was a person I didn't even know who took the time to come and see me graduate. I was so excited and overwhelmed at his interest, I looked past his many flaws. The ones I saw seemed fixable, so we got married. I was 30 pounds overweight.

My husband was a cross country truck driver, so I was alone quite a bit. After 3 years of longing for children, a neighbor introduced me to Jesus. By the grace of God, I found a new family in Christ, but was just a baby Christian with so much to learn.

By the time I was pregnant with our first child, I was 50 pounds overweight. With each of my pregnancies, I lost the baby weight within a week or two, but gained weight in between children. I always imagined being a mother like June Clever from *Leave it to Beaver*. My hair would be fixed, I would have a dress and pearls on, baking sweet treats. No one told me I would be fortunate if I got a shower, that most of my meals would be eaten cold, and I would not sleep through the night for many years. In frustration and weariness, I continued to overeat.

I never thought I had a problem with food. I liked food. Eating something made me feel better. My problem, I thought, was lack of self-control, because I could not resist the temptation of overeat. I had no discipline around food, therefore, I felt like a failure who just couldn't get it right. When I was pregnant with my third child, my husband decided to run off with another woman, leaving me three months pregnant with a one-year old, a three-year old, and no income. Thus, began five years as a single parent learning to trust and rely solely on God. God was a faithful husband and father who took care of all our needs. My church rallied around, but I still struggled with rejection and great brokenness.

A new chapter began when I met my current husband at church. He was the keyboard player and I sang. He truly was (and still is) a gift from God. We married in 1990 and had three more children, losing one in a miscarriage. I had lost weight dating my husband and several more times over the years, losing as much as 80 lbs., but could never maintain the weight loss. I always went back to overeating. I suffered from severe depression during menopause and continued to overeat. My weight topped off at 284 lbs.

About four years ago, the pastor at my church talked about self-medicating. This was a new thought for me. Self-medicating with drugs, alcohol, pornography and yes, food. I realized I might be doing this, so I set up an appointment to meet with her. She took me through the "Seven Steps to Freedom" by Neil Anderson. I went through a lot of inner healing from sexual abuse, abandonment issues and other brokenness. It gave me the strength to go back to Weight Watchers, and I lost about 80 lbs., but once again couldn't maintain it. I tried another program, "Prism," lost 30 lbs., but could not keep the weight off. What was wrong with me? No diet worked for long.

In April 2018, while searching for yet another diet, I saw and read Pam's book, *Sweet Surrender.* It described me. Just like Pam, I was hiding food, snacking after my family went to bed, and I had retrieved food from the garbage. I contacted Pam and had her add me to the Facebook groups. I went to a phone meeting and said I was looking for a sponsor. A precious *Full of Faith* member contacted me, so I tried the Step Easy Food Plan for a few days, but could not give up some of the foods. I was not ready, so I left the program and the groups, but that same *Full of Faith* member continued to sweetly text me from time to time. I thanked her, but told her I had decided to go back to Weight Watchers.

After four months of yo-yo dieting, I was depressed and a mess. My counselor told me I needed an outpatient program. When I asked why, she said, "for food addiction." It felt like a slap in the face! I never in all the years of battling with food thought I could be an addict. I sat in shock! After taking some time to come to grips with this new found revelation, I looked at outpatient programs. With a cost of $3,000 to $5,000 with insurance, there was no way I could do it.

I thought about a 12-step program for overeaters, but I was petrified and really wanted a Christian program. I asked God to help me. In my debate, the same *Full of Faith* member texted me again. At this point, I was at the end of my rope. I had no other choice, but to reach out to Pam. She put me back in the Facebook groups, and since she happened to live about 15 minutes from me, we met face to face.

I began my abstinent journey on September 4th, 2018. I started off with a previous 67 lb. weight loss and have lost an additional 50 lbs. in *Full of Faith*. I still have approximately another 20 lbs. to go. I have not been this weight since high school! I was pre-diabetic, my blood pressure was on the rise, and I had been on a prescription for esophageal reflux, all of which no longer exist. These are small victories in comparison to what I have gained by being a member of *Full of Faith*. I have fellows who walk with me, pray and encourage me, who understand my addiction and have gone before me. I have learned about grace, about feeling feelings and taking them to God. I have learned, and I am continuing to learn, the daily disciplines and the steps that keep me free.

Most importantly, with the food out of the way, not standing between me and God, I am walking closer to God, growing and learning to be loved by Him. It is a good abstinent life, not without trials or temptations, but with all God has provided for me, I am able to walk through the challenging times.

I am thankful for the counselor who told me I am a food addict, to Pam who began the program, to the precious *Full of Faith* member who reached out to me even when I had walked away, to Hilary who lovingly sponsored me at the beginning, to my sponsor who has been invaluable, loving, supportive and full of grace for me when I could not give myself grace, my accountability group, and all the *Full of Faith* members known and unknown who support me through prayers and encouraging words and posts. Elizabeth from MA.

Debra from Canada

Hi, I'm Debra from Canada. My earliest memories include having a sweet tooth. There wasn't a lot of junk food in my house, but when there was, I was obsessed with it. I marveled that people could forget about food and let snacks go stale. I could not.

I was a very sensitive child. Because of this, and a degree of dysfunction in my home, I didn't learn to deal with fears and feelings in a healthy manner. I vacillated between seeking people to validate me and being fiercely self-sufficient. That led to me trusting the wrong people and not reaching out for help to the right people. I didn't know what a healthy relationship looked like. I was full of shame and needed to put up a façade to cover it.

When I was 28, I had all that I thought I needed - marriage, children, financial stability and a home of my own, yet I sensed a void. My concept of God had been that He was keeping score of my deeds and at the end of my life, if I was good enough, I'd be welcomed into heaven. I didn't have much hope. Oh! How thankful I was to be wrong! When I invited Jesus into my heart and my life, he took my deeds and my shame with Him to the cross and gave me His right standing. Jesus paid the penalty for my sins and I felt acceptance, forgiveness, help and hope like never before. A personal relationship with Him started, friendships started. It was a whole new world.

Unfortunately, I still carried a lot of unhealthy habits and misbeliefs - a lot of bondage to self and pride. Still somehow believing I had to pay Jesus back for His sacrifice, I tried to be perfect, but it was a setup for failure. The pain of all that was compounded by the fact that I could not stop overeating. Food was the most acceptable, inexpensive way to manage my anxiety, boredom, anger and fear. I craved foods laden with sugar and flour, and I couldn't stay on any diet for very long. My journals are full of despair and "please forgive me again."

I continued to serve in my Christian community, and I tried to stay connected with the Lord, because He was so winsome and life-giving. Although, in time my faith eroded and I found myself going through the motions, but no longer connecting to the Lord in a personal way. Having a healthy fear of being left to my own devices kept me from turning my back on the Lord completely. I was mad that my life wasn't going the way I wanted. I also feared He would want to address the fact that food had become my idol.

When I was 50, one Sunday morning my Pastor talked about being controlled by the Holy Spirit with passages from Romans 8:6 and Galatians 5:16. I cried. Convicted that I was controlled by circumstances, feelings, food and not the Holy Spirit anymore I booked a meeting with my Pastor. I had been so busy trying to control everything and everybody, that my own needs had been set aside. Instead, I blamed circumstances for my poor choices, bitter attitude and lack of faith. I started counselling and joined a 12-step support group for people who were affected by people with addictions. This renewed my faith and I surrendered to Christ again.

Two years later in 2012, I was at my top weight - over 235 lbs. I had given up and accepted that weight gain, health problems and diminished quality of life were just the way it was going to be. However, God had another plan. As I listened to a 12-step speaker tape one day, I heard someone talking about overeating. Despite my immediate impulse to turn the message off, the Lord gently impressed on me that it was no accident. It was time to open the door to Him in this area of my life. I'm thankful for His faithfulness.

I joined a 12-step fellowship for overeaters and started to apply the 12-steps to my life. I held onto my prideful attitude, because I truly believed I had completed the steps when I became a Christian. Oh, how my Shepherd Jesus must have lovingly chuckled at this sheep's foolishness. When I took the time to write down everything that went into my mouth, it was eye opening. It was a long list. My shell of denial began to crack. Showing my list and committing my food to my sponsor for the first time was very humbling, yet freeing. God's light began to shine on this dark corner at last.

At my first 12-step conference for compulsive overeaters, I heard some people with long term abstinence talk about not eating sugar or flour and weighing and measuring food. My response, "How radical! I could never do that!" So, I set out to find a definition of abstinence that let me eat what I wanted when I wanted in moderation. It brought confusion, not freedom, but it was a start. Preplanning and committing what I was going to eat was a different experience for this girl who was used to going on whims and feelings. Starting to say "no" to myself and working the steps brought some freedom and healing and about a 30 lb. weight loss.

Gradually though I began to feel stuck. I was overcommitted to service and still had cravings and periodic binges. Even preplanning the amounts of sugar, flour and sweeteners didn't help. I could not stay on any food plan for very long. When I told my dear Christian friends, and to be fair, I didn't tell them the goriest details of what I was doing with food, their support and suggestions were wise, but didn't touch my compulsion.

"Take a walk." I knew my sore feet and chafed thighs couldn't out walk the cravings, and I needed to be at home some of the time!

"Pray." Often, I found myself crying and praying while I was ingesting another mouthful of food, and because of the nature of my 12-step group, I couldn't easily bring Christ into any conversations. Frustrated, I began to worry that I would be in a state of semi-recovery, fighting cravings for the rest of my days.

In March 2016, I was introduced to *Full of Faith*. I checked out the website and joined the Facebook groups. Hope grew! It was the best of both worlds - food recovery and faith in Jesus. Worries about it being online rather than face-to-face were allayed with my first phone meeting. I realized the people in *Full of Faith* are real and God is working in and through them. In August, I was blessed with my first *Full of Faith* sponsor. It was God's perfect timing, because I had started to experiment with purging. It was a path to more bondage that was hurting me spiritually, emotionally and physically. Sayings like, "Two wrongs don't make a right," and, "If you ate it, you own it," helped to stop this practice before it got deeply entrenched in my thinking.

With the courage that the Lord provided, I learned to take responsibility for my actions. By going to the Lord and my *Full of Faith* friends to shine a light on each break, I stopped justifying what I was doing and I realized that I needed help. Only God's way works for me.

I had many questions and fears in the beginning. How do I cope with cravings and detox? How do I handle parties, restaurants, leftovers, scoffers, camping and more. By asking and listening, I learned. People are willing to share their experience, strength and hope. The *Full of Faith* community is beautiful.

My willingness was weak. God used the science of food addiction, anger that food manufacturers used addictive substances to sell products, and my food history to increase my willingness. The Bright Line Eating intro videos, Food Addiction Institute.org, Pam's book (the first edition of *Sweet Surrender*) and the *Full of Faith* group helped me accept that I was a food addict who needed a structured recovery program with lots of accountability. For me this can be called a journey out of shame and lies.

In July 2017, I joined an accountability group whose focus was working every tool every day. Another huge blessing! I've learned that the tools do not keep me abstinent. They create a space in my life for the Lord to come in and work.

By the fall of 2017, I was struggling with increasing breaks and slips. I was getting right back, but I was playing with fire, so to speak. I justified these slips because I was approaching goal weight, and I was in emotional upheaval over hurtful choices of loved ones. The culprit - I still had food in my tool box to numb me when I was feeling strong feelings.

In time I learned to be open and honest. I then found hope, help and healing. Listening to food addicts' experiences taught me that I was not alone. When I was struggling to maintain my abstinence, another food addict suggested doing a 4th step inventory in a different way. I did it and was surprised to see hidden truths. Writing out the thoughts that lead to the first bite helped, too. Previously, I believed "it won't matter." Well, it sure did. By making the commitment to remove spontaneous eating from my toolbox, whether abstinent food or not, meant I had to work the tools (the daily disciplines of the program) and the 12-steps as if my life depended on it. I heard "God and abstinence are the most important thing to me, without exception." Actively participating in formal step studies kept me grounded and allowed me to grow. I had to learn healthy self-care, boundaries, gratitude and many other things. I'm still learning! Dec 18, 2017 was my last break, and I marvel that it happened before my most challenging holiday.

Now my journals are full of hope and wise insights, less despair. Spiritually, my faith and trust in the Lord is growing because the barriers between the Lord and myself are coming down. Physically, I never imagined that this lifestyle would become automatic. I no longer miss my binge foods, cravings have become rare, I have lost all my excess weight (over 100 lbs.), and kept it off. My blood pressure is normal for the first time in decades, and I don't have to keep having my liver checked because of fatty liver disease. Emotionally, I'm more resilient, confident and have deeper, more peaceful relationships.

Recovery from food addiction is more than not eating certain foods for me. It is a lifestyle of letting God reign in all areas of my life and letting him change me step by step to be more like Christ.

When I joined *Full of Faith*, I was encouraged to write my vision for recovery. With a tiny mustard seed of faith, I wrote: "I am seeking the Lord first thing in the morning, feeding on His Word to learn more of His will and ways. When emotions and circumstances are uncomfortable, my heart turns to Jesus and my ears to hear the voice of my King, not to food or the lies of the enemy. I am letting Him fight my battles, trusting that He will never leave me or forsake me. I embrace His discipline because He is transforming me. I am saved for a wonderful purpose. I am following a food plan – not eating sugar, flour, sweetener and volume. I am free. He is growing this sapling into a lovely tree!" Debra from Canada

Cheryl from CA
FROM HOPELESSNESS TO HOPE

In testimony to God's amazing and healing grace, I would like to share my story of experience, strength and hope. The Lord led me to recovery and has been with me every step of the way.

Today I am 70 years old. I am much healthier physically, emotionally and spiritually than I was at 50. I came into 12-step recovery at 58 in 2007 weighing 308 pounds, wearing size 22/24. I saw my top weight, 314 pounds, on the scale of a personal trainer I had hired to help me with my weight. During an 18-month period in 12-step recovery, I lost 180 pounds, averaging 10 pounds per month. I have maintained a normal-sized body for over 10 years, wearing size 6/8.

At the time I entered my first 12-step program from food addiction, I was on three different blood pressure medications. I was pre-diabetic and had plantar fasciitis. It was extremely painful to walk. I had to use a walking stick if I needed to walk any distance because my knees would give out; I would fall and couldn't get up. I had sleep apnea and was using a bi-pap machine. I was also taking anti-depressants and anti-anxiety medications, even though I was in denial and didn't think I needed them. My therapist thought it might help my "overeating problem". She thought that maybe my uncontrollable eating was caused by stress or anxiety. Today I take no prescription medications and walk without assistance.

As a child I loved desserts and high fat foods. My mother was always concerned about her weight and closely monitored mine, so I learned early on to sneak sweet, starchy and high-fat foods. I was fairly active in my youth, so my overeating did not appear on my body until I was 22 years old. During my first pregnancy, I gained 60 pounds.

After my daughter's birth, I began my life of roller coaster dieting, using every diet program or weight-loss method on the market - Weight Watchers, Jenny Craig, Diet Center, hypnotherapy, in-patient lifestyle programs, hiring a personal trainer, and even colon cleansing. Each time I tried one of these programs, I would think, "This is it. I'll do it this time." I remember my wedding ring getting tighter, but because I believed I was going to lose weight, I ignored the warnings until my finger was in extreme pain and it was necessary to have a jeweler cut the ring off my finger.

At 30, I weighed 200 pounds. By the time I was 34, after my son's birth, I was over 260 pounds. I continued to struggle with morbid obesity for another 25 years. There was nothing that would or could stop me from eating uncontrollably. Even though my father had died from a heart attack, as had both of his parents, and I had high blood pressure, heading towards a stroke or heart attack, I could not stop myself.

I went to one specific in-patient lifestyle program several different times over a five-year period. In that program I continued to have tests to monitor my heart, because I told myself if I saw a poor test result that would encourage me to stop eating. However, I ignored and buried any tests results that showed there might be a problem, and I continued to overeat.

When I was pregnant with my second child, because of how large I was, I didn't even know I was pregnant until I felt movement in my stomach. I rushed to the doctor because I thought something was horribly wrong with me (another example of my denial). He performed an ultrasound and told me I was pregnant. Soon after, he placed me on bed rest and diagnosed me with toxemia. At that time, he told me that both myself and my baby could die if I continued eating the way I was. Although I stayed in bed, I continued to eat that way until my son was born a few months later, by caesarian and not at full-term. Thankfully, although premature, he had no continuing health problems.

At 58 my life consisted of isolating myself to the best of my ability. I had stopped going to church, because I didn't want to go out in public. My focus was on satisfying myself with food, rather than turning to God. I had a home office. After my employees left for the day, my outings consisted of going to drive-thru restaurants and stockpiling my food for the night, or I would have food delivered to my door and sit in front of the television eating until bedtime.

My therapist heard about a food addiction recovery program from a family member and suggested I try it. When

I walked through the door of my first 12-step meeting, about 80 people surrounded me as a newcomer and shared their stories. Love and hope washed over me. I had a true "spiritual awakening." I saw and heard the miracles of recovery, looked at pictures and soon realized I am a food addict. If I just did what these people did, I would receive what they had. My initial focus was a normal-sized body. They told me to find a sponsor who has what I wanted, and ask them how it was achieved. I wanted to be thin, so that's what I looked for in a sponsor. Today I see that I came for the vanity, and stayed for the sanity.

Thankfully, the Lord led me to a sponsor who taught me a disciplined way of life, beginning with a food plan. Beyond that, I started to develop some integrity by reading to her my daily food plan, and eating only what I had committed. She taught me the importance of beginning and ending each day with prayer (in the morning asking God to help me have an abstinent day, and at bedtime thanking Him for my abstinent day), 30-minutes of quiet time each morning, going to at least three committed weekly meetings, making daily calls to three other food addicts (calling at least one or two each day who had long-term abstinence, so I could learn from them how they lived free and clean), reading from the AA Big Book and a daily meditation book and doing service (giving back what I had so generously been given).

A few months after beginning my recovery, at the suggestion of my sponsor, I started attending an AWOL (A Way of Life), an in-depth study of the 12-steps in a closed group of people fully committed to abstinence. Participating in the AWOL helped me begin to learn how to turn both my addiction and my life over to the care of God. Working through the 12-steps continually is how God has guided me, and continues to guide me today, to have not only physical healing, but also spiritual and emotional recovery.

When my husband and I retired in 2013, I asked God to lead me to a ministry that would provide me with opportunities to help and encourage others, while strengthening my relationship with Him. By God's grace, in 2016, I was led to *Full of Faith*. Because it is a Christian 12-step program, I am experiencing God's love, grace and mercy by reading, applying and sharing God's Word at meetings and with members one to one. In *Full of Faith*, we study the 12-steps from a biblical perspective, using *The Twelve Steps for Christians* and *The Life Recovery Bible*.

God has answered my prayers in so many ways. In *Full of Faith*, I do a lot of "love and service," and I am a member of the leadership team of overseers. Today, as long as I continue to keep my eyes on Him, I continue to move forward toward the plans he has for me, one day at a time. Cheryl from CA

Monica from NH
For more than 50 years, I was held captive by my addiction to food. I tried diet after diet and don't ever remember a time when I was at peace with my weight or body size. I lost and gained weight over and over again (mostly gained) and was unable to find stability for my mind or body. I knew I had a problem with food and was continually trying to find a way to eat like "normal" people. In 2015, through a Google search, I found *Full of Faith*. I tried to implement some of the suggestions made, because I weighed over 170 pounds, but with my limited willingness, I only lost about 10 pounds in over a year, and I was still out of control and miserable most of the time.

In July of 2016 I came back to *Full of Faith* with a changed heart. It was like coming home. In August 2016, I humbled myself and let God and others help me, and then lost more than 50 more pounds. I am learning that living in freedom has very little to do with what I am eating or not eating, but has everything to do with surrender and sanity.

Addiction can be defined as an allergy of the body and an obsession of the mind. A person caught in addiction has the delusion that someday they will break out and tame the beast that is ruling over them. Being caught in addiction was especially painful for this Christian who knew she belonged to Jesus, but was not experiencing freedom. That was where I found myself for years and years. Romans 7:15 describes the struggle, " For what I do is not the good I want to do, no, the evil I do not want to do, this I keep on doing." Addiction had me locked in insanity which can be defined as doing the same thing over and over again and expecting different results.

Romans 7:24 was my theme verse, "What a wretched man I am! Who will rescue me from this body of death?" I thought Jesus would, but it was just not happening.
When struggling with my addiction, in addict-like fashion, I had all kinds of excuses, rationalizations, and justifications. I was like the Pharisee praying in Luke 18:11,"The Pharisee stood by himself and prayed: 'God, I thank you that I am not like other people--robbers, evildoers, adulterers--or even like this tax collector." My idea of an addict was a skid-row bum, and that was not me. I knew that I was off in my thinking and behavior, but I still thought I was not that bad. But my own desperation to be free finally led me to realize that I was not going to beat my addiction my way or by myself. I had to be the tax collector, bow my head and say, "God have mercy on me, a sinner."

Addiction took me places that I never wanted to go and accepting that I was an addict and could not fix myself was very painful. To surrender and admit that my life was unmanageable by me made me feel like I was going into exile or being punished by God. But I was beaten; I was sick and tired of being sick and tired.

When I finally joined *Full of Faith*, when I was willing to humble myself and message Pam to say, "Sign me up," I began doing my one percent. God has been faithfully showing up to do the other 99 percent. Instead of waking up saying, "Good God, it's morning," and knowing by ten

213

o'clock, or even earlier, that all of my vows, plans, schemes, and resolve would be used up, I can say, "Good morning, God!" and surrender to do His will just for today.

I was afraid to see what kind of crazies were in *Full of Faith*, but I now consider the members some of my nearest and dearest friends. We love, pray for and support each other moment by moment, day by day. We practice honesty and keep no secrets. God does for us what we could not do for ourselves. I was terrified of failure after failing so many times, but by joining a group of people who share my common problem, I am no longer alone.

One of my favorite lessons in recovery is that Jesus really is the answer, and He really loves me and paid dearly for my freedom. Once, on one of the daily phone meetings, someone was speaking about John the Baptist. In Luke 7, John is in prison, and he sends his disciples to ask Jesus, "Are you the one who is to come or should we expect someone else?" I was struck by this question. I had known that I had Jesus, but was still looking for someone or something else. Jesus told John's messengers, "Go back and report to John what you have seen and heard. The blind receive sight, the lame walk, those who have leprosy are cleansed, the deaf hear, the dead are raised, and the good news is proclaimed to the poor. Blessed is anyone who does not stumble on account of me."

I had infirmities, but with Jesus and recovery, I am being given daily freedom. Because of recovery and the freedom God has given me, I now live the miracle. Instead of imagining my own power and tripping over Jesus, I can get out of the way and acknowledge Him as Lord.

Instead of struggling to fix myself, I can accept the help offered. 1 Corinthians 10 :13 tells us that, "Nothing has seized us that is not common to man." I like the word "seized," because that gives a good harsh word for what addiction does; it holds me in a death grip. Jesus and Christians who share a common affliction are available to walk the walk with me. There is no need to battle it out alone.

Admitting that I had a problem was difficult, but it has turned out to be one of the greatest blessings of my life. God's strength is perfected in weakness, and knowing I am powerless is the absolute beginning of healing. God has shown Himself to be powerful in my life and in the lives of others with whom I share the journey. 2 Corinthians 12:9 says, "Most gladly therefore I will rather glory in my infirmities that the power of Christ may rest upon me!"

I invite you to follow His lead. Help is here, and He can do more than we can ask or imagine. At this writing, I have now been living in freedom one day at a time for almost three years. I learned that being a food addict is not a curse, but a blessing. I get to live in fellowship with others who share my struggle, and God has turned my misery into a mission for which I am grateful.

> LORD Our God, other lords besides you have ruled over us, but your name alone do we honor. (Isaiah 26:13)

Monica from NH

Sonia from CA

I am a food addict; I am completely powerless over sugar, flour and quantities. I am grateful today that I know this truth about myself. I began my 12-step recovery from food addiction in 2004. I was 37 years old and weighed 275.5 pounds. My weight was continuously climbing, even though I was always searching for the newest diet to try.

I come from a family with a long history of struggling with obesity and alcoholism. Food was my drug of choice, but alcohol was another substance that I didn't know how to moderate. One is too many, a thousand is not enough. I never ate food or drank alcohol in moderation. I always ate until my stomach ached and drank until my head started to spin, or I went too far and got physically sick.

Body size and low self-esteem were problems early on. I was around ten years old when I remember feeling different - fat, not smart enough, not good enough. I felt I didn't fit in. I lived in fear. My father was killed when I was one year old, leaving my mother with four young children. We had a lot of people living in our home over the years. I was, most of the time, not in a safe environment and no one spoke of what was going on all around us.

Food was my solace, my escape, my comfort and my friend. From a young age, I started stealing and sneaking food, primarily sweet treats and snack foods. I didn't recognize shame at the time, but later identified the feeling. I was very sneaky, not wanting others to see me getting more and more. I remember eating food off others' plates, eating cold, stale or bad tasting food just because I felt a need to fill myself - to numb from thoughts of fear, confusion, remorse. I know now it was that God-shaped hole I kept trying to fill with food.

Growing up, I was taught religious beliefs and practices, but my relationship with God was not grounded in understanding God's Word. I would pray and ask God for help, then forget. I was scared because I felt I was bad and that God was angry at me. I isolated a lot, had a lot of negative, self-destructive thinking. Today, I know my God never thought of me that way.

I started dieting at 12 or 13 years of age. My whole family struggled with weight, so my mother would buy diet pills, powders and shakes to try and help everyone lose weight. I tried diet clubs, magazines, books, always searching for the magic diet that was going to melt off the weight without giving up my favorite foods. Each diet typically lasted a handful of hours to a few days.

Sad to say, my husband and our three sons experienced the effects of my being face down in the food. My moods were all over the place, because food controlled me. My mind was completely wrapped around what I was going to eat and where and how I was I going to get it, which was always followed by regret of eating too much and wondering how I was going to finally lose weight. I was so preoccupied with these thoughts that I became irritable and intolerant of people around me, especially the ones that needed my care and attention. My family felt it the most. I raged, because I had so much fear and insecurity.

Our finances were greatly affected by my wanting/needing more of something. In time, the food stopped working. I still ate large amounts of sugar, flour, salt and greasy foods, but it wasn't enough, so I picked up other addictions, always looking for something to make me feel better. Taking antidepressants numbed the feelings that surfaced. Without much hope, I went to a therapist and blamed everything and everyone for my misery and struggles, not recognizing I played a role in each situation.

Another distraction became buying things we could not afford, which brought us financial trouble. I shopped and spent money without thought, got lost at the mall, escaping from my reality and responsibilities. But with all this, I'm grateful. My experiences brought me to the place of being bloodied, beaten and desperate. I finally admitted I was completely out of control, nothing was working.

At my first 12-step meeting for food addiction, I heard people sharing their experience, strength and hope. I was amazed. Many had lost (released) large amounts of weight and kept it off. They had joy in their lives. Their relationships and finances were better. Many more witnessed how surrendering and willingness brought freedom from the obsession with food. It got my attention, and I started my journey in recovery shortly thereafter.

I joined *Full of Faith* in June of 2018, already at goal weight, having lost over 130 pounds and keeping it off for over 14 years in my first 12-step recovery group. My recovery has definitely been a journey that continues. I often say I feel like a toddler - learning, making mistakes, accepting help. My journey since coming into *Full of Faith* has given me the gift of a deeper, more personal relationship with Jesus. I know that my success and recovery is by God's grace. I can't, but God can.

Surrendering and admitting I'm powerless, I work the steps as a way of life. I have a sponsor, connect with other food addicts, pray, meditate, attend meetings and practice the tools of the program to the best of my ability one day at a time. The more I work the program, the more freedom I have around the food, more neutrality to its presence.

I love the Christian aspect of *Full of Faith*, as it has brought my recovery to a whole new level, a much deeper love for the Lord and a truly grateful heart for all the gifts He has given me in recovery. I have a community of like-minded people, all trying to abstain from dieting and overeating one day at a time.

My life today is changed. I praise God that I can say I love myself, and I love and enjoy the people in my life. I look forward to continuing my journey with my community in *Full of Faith* and I thank God for all the blessings I have today. I don't have to eat today to feel better. I ask God for help, I weigh and measure my food, and I use the tools of the program. The program works! Sonia from CA

Nancy from CO

"You chose me. You're all these people: you're the mother, you're the designer, you're the teacher, you're the worker, you're my lover," said my husband of thirty-six years as we snuggled one morning.

All my life I wanted to be loved and accepted like that, but for many years my worth and value was wrapped around the size of my body. Therefore, I tried to fix myself by losing weight. I believed if I could just lose weight and be skinny, then all the good things, all the things I longed for, would come true in my life. It seemed simple. If I ate less, the weight would come off, but I proved over and over again that I had no control over the amount of food I ate. I used food as a comforter and a friend. I used food to hide from life. It provided an escape from reality.

What was wrong with me?

When I was 16, I went to church camp and accepted Jesus Christ as my Lord and Savior. This was, and still is, the most miraculous thing that has happened to me in my lifetime.

With my newfound faith, I prayed fervently for God to take this weight problem away from me, but nothing changed, so I spent the next 40+ years trying every weight-loss program on the planet. Still, no lasting success until, at the exact right time, God led me to Pam's book, *Sweet Surrender*. During Christmas break in 2015, I read and cried over every word. What a revelation! I identified with everything Pam talked about, from trying to control her food to trying to control her life. The most amazing thing to me was how she had incorporated the Twelve Steps of Alcoholics Anonymous with her Christian faith. I had been a leader in a Christian weight loss group for several years, so I knew that it was possible to do so, but in her book, she made it sound so simple. I emailed her and became a member of the *Full of Faith* Facebook groups.

It was sweet relief to be part of a community of Christian food addicts, who had found a solution - God's solution. I read all of the posts and all of the references. I educated myself about what it meant to be a food addict, and I found a food sponsor. Since February 18, 2016, I have been abstinent from flour, sugar, sweeteners (both artificial and natural), caffeine, dairy products and for the most part, grains. I have a healthy food plan that supplies adequate protein, carbohydrates and fats. I plan what I am going to eat each day and then I eat what I planned. It is not deprivation, but freedom.

My attitude and behavior began to change the first time I walked through the intense 12-steps study found in the Big Book, *Alcoholics Anonymous,* with my peers. I discovered that I have the disease of compulsive overeating and I am a food addict. The most amazing discovery was the fact that I have a two-part illness: I have an allergy of the body to certain substances. Whenever I ingest them, I am biochemically driven to continue eating them. In the Big Book, this is called the "phenomenon of craving."

Finding out about the second part of the illness was even more telling for me. It is called the "obsession of the mind." The Big Book tells me that I am powerless over that obsession and that no matter what I do, I will keep returning to the food. I knew that was true from my personal experience!

The best news is that, "There is One who has all of the power, and that One is God." So, here I discovered in the Big Book that the solution to my problem was to be found in God all the time. By working through the Steps as written in the Big Book as a way of life, I have found that the Promises on pages 83 and 84 have come true in my life. Here's my rendition of them:

- If I am persistent in pursuing the 12-step way of life, I will be amazed at how quickly I see and feel changes taking place in my attitude and my behavior.

- I will enjoy a newfound freedom and a newfound happiness.

- I will not regret my past, nor wish to keep secrets or embellish the truth.
- I will understand serenity and will experience peace.

- No matter how bad my life gets, God will use my experience to help others.

- I will no longer feel sorry for myself, be selfish, self-seeking or manipulative.

- I will not be afraid of anyone.

- The way I look at everything and feel about everything will change.

- I will no longer fear being in financial ruin or expect a financial crisis.

- I will know how to handle situations that seem overwhelming at first glance.

- I will realize that God is doing for me what I could not do for myself.

Now, my life is good. Food is neutral, it doesn't call to me, and I have a new relationship with God. After losing my excess weight, I realized that losing weight wasn't the most important thing. The most important thing was gaining a new relationship with God, Jesus Christ, that I needed all along. Today I have a husband who loves me, not because I am thin and look good, but because God has changed me. He has made me a new person. The Big Book tells me that my purpose in life is to serve God and serve others. Love and service is helping others because people have helped me. I have surrendered my food and my life to God, and God has given me a whole new life. Nancy from CO

Bibliography

Alcoholics Anonymous, third edition, New York: Alcoholics Anonymous World Service, 1976.

Friends in Recovery, *The Twelve Steps for Christians,* Revised Edition, California: RPI Publishing, Inc., 1994.

Sheppard, Kay, *Food Addiction: The Body Knows,* Revised Edition, Florida: Health Communications, Inc., l993.

The Amplified Bible, Michigan: Zondervan Corporation and California: The Lockman Foundation, 1987.

The Holy Bible, New International Version, Michigan: Zondervan Publishing House and International Bible Society, l984.

The Holy Bible, The New Living Translation, Illinois: Tyndale House Publishers, Inc., 1996.

The Living Bible, Illinois: Tyndale House Publishers, Inc., 1971.

The excerpts from the book, *Alcoholics Anonymous* and the Twelve Steps of Alcoholics Anonymous, as adapted by adding biblical scriptures are reprinted with an adaptation of biblical scriptures with permission of Alcoholics Anonymous World Services, Inc. (A.A.W.S.) Permission to reprint these excerpts and reprint the adaptation of the Twelve Steps does not mean that A.A.W.S. has reviewed or approved the contents of this publication, or that A.A.W.S. necessarily agrees with the views expressed herein. A.A. is a program of recovery from alcoholism only – use of the Twelve Steps in connection with programs and activities which are patterned after A.A., but which address other problems, or in any other non-A.A. context, does not imply otherwise. Additionally,

223

while A.A. is a spiritual program, A.A. is not a religious program. Thus, A.A. is not affiliated or allied with any sect, denomination, or specific religious belief.

Statement of Faith

I believe in...

...**One God,** the Father, Son and Holy Spirit, who created all things by His almighty power and is in control of all things.

...**The Bible**, which is God's Word, and tells us all we need to know about what we should believe and how we should live.

...**Man**, who was created perfect in the image of God, but who through disobedience became a slave of sin and liable to God's justice.

...**Jesus Christ**, the eternal Son of God, who became man, lived a sinless life and died in our place, taking away our guilt; who rose physically from the dead and is alive and reigning in heaven today as Lord of all; who will one day come again to this world and judge all people, condemning those who are impenitent and unbelieving, and taking to glory with Him those who have truly believed in Him.

...**The Holy Spirit**, who works in the hearts of sinners, enabling them to believe in Jesus Christ and to repent of their sins, and who is a living reality in the lives of those who are true believers.

...**The Forgiveness of Sin**, which comes about as God's free and undeserved gift through the death of Jesus Christ and is received only through faith in Him.

...**The Church,** which is the world-wide community of all who truly believe in the Lord Jesus Christ.

The 12 Steps of Alcoholics Anonymous

1. We admitted we were powerless over alcohol—that our lives had become unmanageable.

2. Came to believe that a Power greater than ourselves could restore us to sanity.

3. Made a decision to turn our will and our lives over to the care of God as we understood Him.

4. Made a searching and fearless moral inventory of ourselves.

5. Admitted to God, to ourselves, and to another human being the exact nature of our wrongs.

6. Were entirely ready to have God remove all these defects of character.

7. Humbly asked Him to remove our shortcomings.

8. Made a list of all persons we had harmed, and became willing to make amends to them all.

9. Made direct amends to such people wherever possible, except when to do so would injure them or others.

10. Continued to take personal inventory and when we were wrong promptly admitted it.

11. Sought through prayer and meditation to improve our conscious contact with God as we understood Him, praying only for knowledge of His will for us and the power to carry that out.

12. Having had a spiritual awakening as the result of these steps, we tried to carry this message to alcoholics, and to practice these principles in all our affairs.

Made in the USA
Coppell, TX
06 April 2022

76112856R00142